Pembroke Branch Tel. 6689575

THE

YOGA

—HANDBOOK—

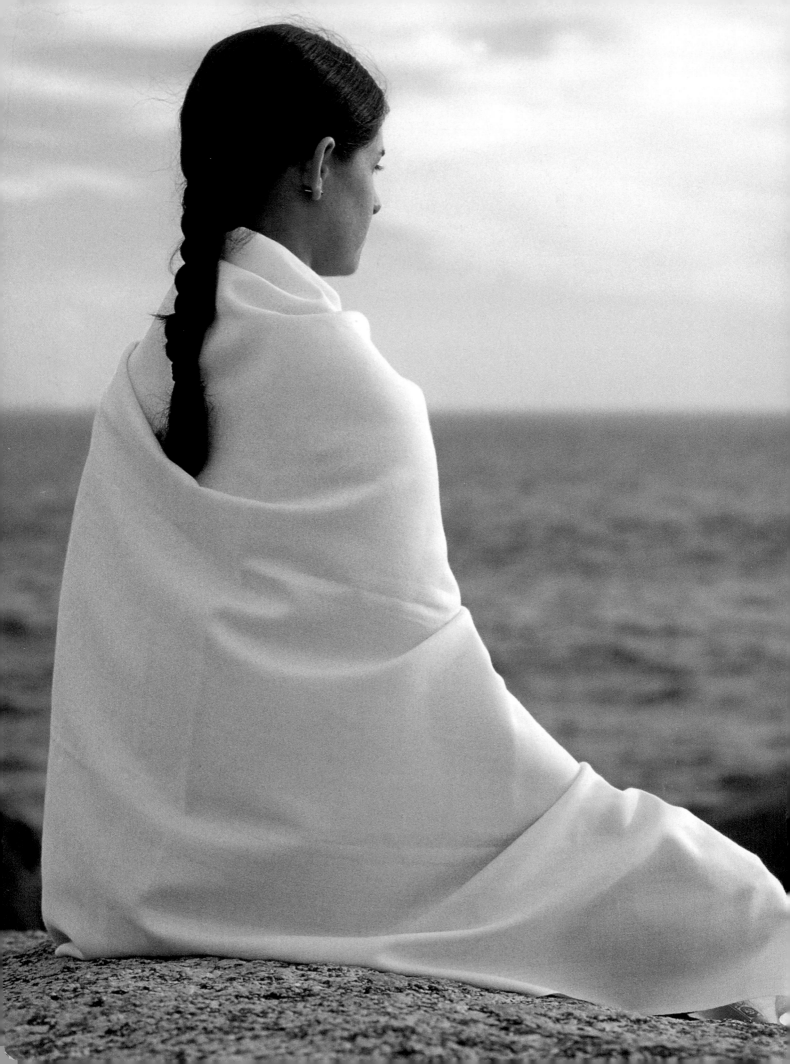

THE
YOGA
HANDBOOK

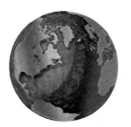

NEW HOLLAND

Noa Belling

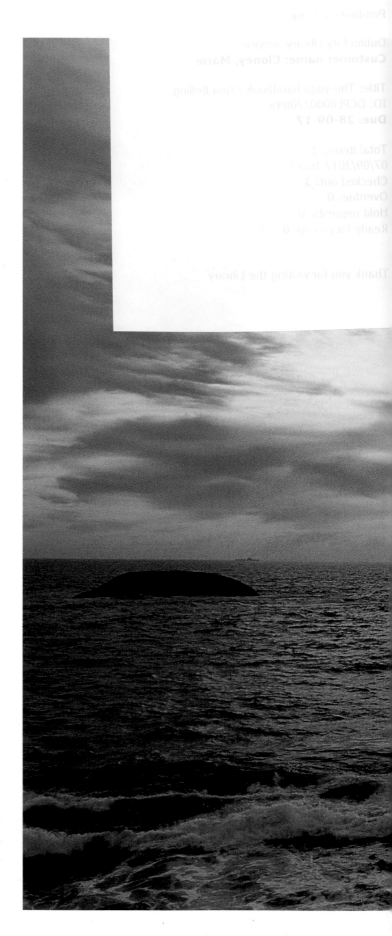

First published in 2001
This edition published in 2008 by
New Holland Publishers (UK) Ltd
London • Cape Town • Sydney • Auckland

Garfield House, 86–88
Edgware Road, London, W2 2EA
United Kingdom

80 McKenzie Street
Cape Town 8001
South Africa

Unit 1, 66 Gibbes Street
Chatswood, NSW 2067
Australia

218 Lake Road
Northcote, Auckland
New Zealand

ISBN 978 1 84537 935 3

PUBLISHER: Mariëlle Renssen
MANAGING EDITORS: Claudia Dos Santos, Mari Roberts
MANAGING ART EDITOR: Peter Bosman
EDITOR: Gail Jennings
DESIGNER: Daniël Jansen van Vuuren
PHOTOGRAPHER: Ryno Reyneke
ILLUSTRATORS: Linda Strydom, Daniël Jansen van Vuuren
PRODUCTION: Myrna Collins
INDEXER AND PROOFREADER: Sean Fraser
CONSULTANTS: David Jacobs (SA), Simon Low (UK)

Reproduction by Unifoto (Pty) Ltd
Printed and bound in Malaysia
by Times Offset (M) Sdn Bhd
6 8 10 9 7 5

Contents

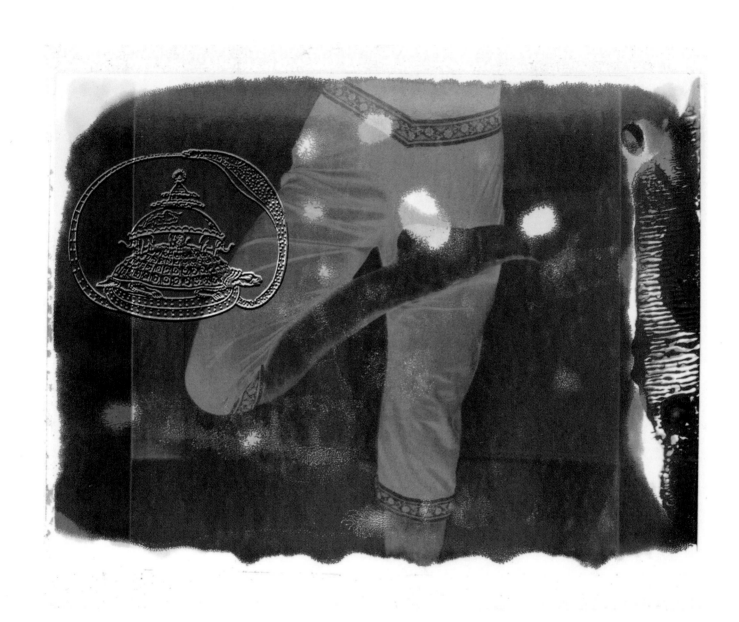

CHAPTER 1

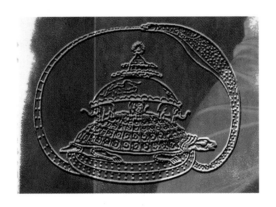

AN INTRODUCTION TO YOGA

An introduction to Yoga

The word Yoga is derived from the Sanskrit language and means to unite or to harmonize. In other words, Yoga means working towards a level where the activities of the mind and body function together harmoniously.

Yoga also refers to the union between the individual and something greater, whether it is called God, the Divine or anything else. Nevertheless, Yoga does not represent or promote any particular religion; it is a system that aims to help people achieve their full potential and a heightened consciousness. This is achieved through age-old techniques, accessible to anyone who is interested. These techniques work towards the development of every human faculty: physical, emotional, mental and spiritual.

The science of Yoga is vast and has been divided into several branches, and each branch focuses on a different means of achieving union with the Divine or the greatness of human potential. The idea of many branches is to be able to accommodate all types of people. The main branches may be described as follows:

- Hatha Yoga works through the mastery of the body and breath. This is the most practical of the branches of Yoga, and is the best known Yoga in the West. It involves a system of exercise that trains through physical postures, breathing and relaxation techniques. These techniques benefit the nervous system, glands and vital organs. The aim is to promote vibrant health and to tap into the body's latent energy reserves. Some say its aim is also to prepare the body for Raja Yoga, which works on consciousness itself, although even Hatha Yoga on its own exerts an integrating and calming influence over the mind.
- Raja Yoga works through the mastery of the mind. This branch involves mental disciplines to work towards mastering consciousness and stilling the thoughts of the mind. This is considered to be the royal path of Yoga, as the Sanskrit word Raja means 'king' or 'supreme'.
- Jnana Yoga works through knowledge (ultimately self-knowledge) and involves the study of your preferred scriptures and meditation.
- Bhakti Yoga works through love and devotion. This branch often involves devotion to a preferred deity, guru or prophet. The disciplines of this path include the expression of total devotion through their preferred rites, rituals, singing and praising.
- Karma Yoga works through selfless action and service.
- Mantra Yoga works through vocal or mental repetition of sacred sounds. This is thought to alter consciousness through the repetition of certain syllables, words or phrases, referred to as mantras. When chanted rhythmically, it is called 'japa'.
- Laya or Kundalini Yoga works through awakening and raising the body's latent psychic nerve-force (kundalini) through several energy centres (chakras). This involves a combination of Hatha Yoga techniques, mainly focusing on breath suspension and intense meditation practice.
- Tantric Yoga, in its most common application, works through the harnessing of sexual energy. It involves the control over the sexual energies and, although it may be practised alone, prepares for the union of male and female, in order to achieve union with the Divine.

The focus of this handbook is on Hatha Yoga, although a small Raja Yoga component is included as an introduction to meditation.

In Yoga, the body is seen as a tool for the mind to be able to make contact with the world. Raja Yoga deals with the training of self-mastery: of the mind over the body, and the will over the mind. Thus the practice of Hatha Yoga is enhanced by Raja Yoga.

WHAT IS HATHA YOGA?

In the compound word Hatha, 'ha' means sun and 'tha' means moon. This refers to the balance of male and female, day and night, positive and negative, yin and yang, hot and cold, or any other opposite, yet balancing pairs.

When this concept is applied, it could refer to bringing the two sides of the body into a state of balance, through the development of equal strength and flexibility on both sides. It could also refer to bringing the two hemispheres of the brain into balanced functioning, so that the logical, mathematical side and the creative, intuitive side are encouraged to function harmoniously and equally efficiently.

In Yoga, the flow of the breath through the right nostril is called the sun breath; the flow through the left nostril is called the moon breath. Breath regulation in some form is central to all Hatha Yoga practice.

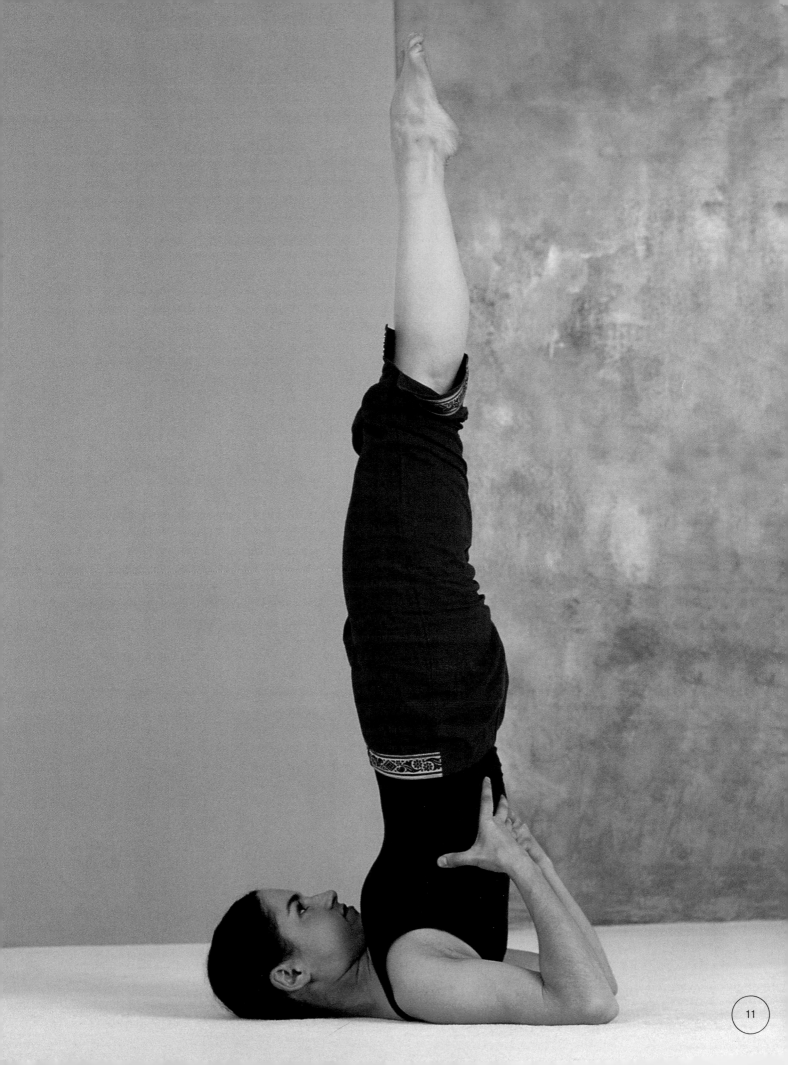

THE BENEFITS OF YOGA

Yoga is a system of personal growth and development. In life, whether we realize it or not, each person strives for happiness and wellbeing. However, all too often the paths we take to do so are more destructive than good. Quick fixes are chosen over long-lasting, healthy options that require some degree of effort.

Wellbeing and happiness

Yoga is a system of health maintenance that is long lasting and cultivates a sense of happiness and fulfilment. It achieves this by teaching how to tap into inner energy reserves and generate health and happiness from within. True happiness cannot be bought – it is the result of a life-long investment in health.

Yoga enhances the health and youthfulness of the body and clarity of the mind. Thus a regular practice can help to counter general physical decline due to ageing, negligent use of the body and/or the accumulation of excess tension.

Enhanced body awareness

Yoga is a means of becoming more familiar with your body (the inner and outer landscape), as the different Yoga postures are together designed to benefit every anatomical structure, system and organ in the body.

This process of learning how to assist the body in its healthy functioning can be empowering. It teaches the participant how to make changes in the body, mind and emotional state and therefore take control of their life and health (physically, mentally, emotionally and spiritually).

Stress relief and prevention

Life today is fast-paced, competitive and stressful, although not all stress is detrimental. Moderate stress can be uplifting and invigorating.

Nevertheless, when the demands placed upon us greatly exceed our habitual levels of performance or coping (whether they are physical, emotional or mental), we suffer discomfort and strain and the body's defences become overworked and exhausted. Side effects include frustration, muscular tension (resulting particularly in back problems), depression, anxiety,

shortness of breath and problems of concentration. Yoga works to free the body from these symptoms of stress. Firstly, deep relaxation training focuses on the body, the mind and the emotions – these skills are effective in countering many symptoms of stress.

Secondly, flexibility exercises are helpful in preventing or alleviating muscular tension.

Thirdly, the use of controlled, deep breathing while executing postures helps to counter any shortness or irregularity of breathing associated with stress. It also helps to achieve and maintain a state of calmness and emotional stability, as the breath is closely linked to emotions and the state of mind.

Finally, the training of Raja Yoga meditation, especially when added to other Yoga techniques, enhances patience and clarity of mind and improves the ability to cope with stress.

Why Yoga rather than other forms of exercise?

Many forms of exercise aim to develop only the superficial muscles of the body and often neglect flexibility training.

Yoga provides a comprehensive system of exercise that stretches, strengthens, tones, helps to align and improves the health of the entire body. Yoga also develops a state of mental calmness and emotional stability. Thus Yoga is unique in that it focuses on the entire body and mind.

Many conventional forms of exercise serve purely aesthetic purposes. According to Yoga philosophy, though, health is first an inner state. This means that the health of the nerves, glands and vital organs determines how healthy a person looks and feels.

What also sets Yoga apart from many other forms of exercise is the co-ordination of breath with each posture and movement. Working with the breath in a conscious manner brings the mind's attention into the present, to the task at hand. This helps to prevent injuries as it ensures that the focus is on the exercise being done. It benefits the functioning of the lungs and the entire respiratory system and increases lung capacity, and it also one's ability to concentrate.

Yoga is non-competitive, which sets it apart from many other sporting and recreational activities. It allows each person to work within personal limits.

Yoga is suitable for all ages and levels of fitness, as it can be a very gentle form of exercise, or it can be rigorous, depending on the practitioner.

It is important to note that regular Yoga practice can be combined with gym or cardiovascular training programmes, sports, dance or any other activity.

Why use this book about Yoga?

- It offers step-by-step guidance with clear progression from beginner to advanced.
- It is suitable for all ages and levels of fitness, as it offers a number of versions of each posture, from the simplest to the most advanced version.
- It does not promote any school of Yoga or religion.
- It introduces basic elements common to most schools of Yoga.
- It focuses on the physical, mental, emotional and spiritual benefits of the various postures.
- It points out cautions for specific postures.
- It can be used in addition to attending Yoga classes, in order to allow you to practise safely at home, familiarize yourself with the names and execution of the postures and speed up your rate of improvement.

How to use this book

- When a sequence of postures is presented, each step is numbered from 1 onwards.
- When options or unrelated steps are presented, they are ordered from A onwards.

Health, according to Yoga philosophy, is made up of regular exercise in the form of physical posturing, proper breathing, sufficient rest and relaxation, meditation to cultivate mental focus and serenity, positive thinking and a healthy, balanced diet. Yoga is one of the few systems that encompasses all of these components.

HEALTH, THE YOGA WAY

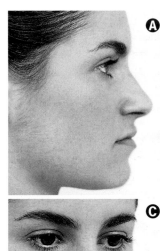
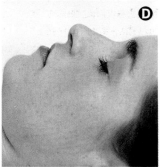
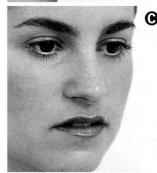
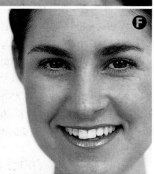
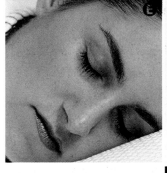
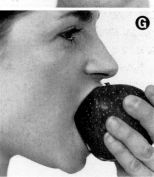
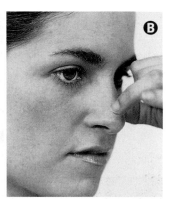

A Posture
B Breathing
C Meditation
D Relaxation
E Sleep
F Positive thinking
G Healthy diet

A history of Yoga

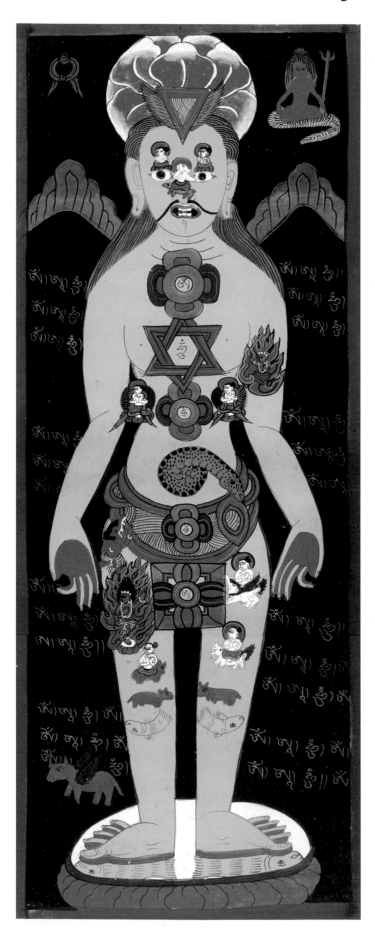

The Sanskrit terms

Translation from Sanskrit to English is a tricky task. Sanskrit terms have been interpreted in many different ways by many different people, thus a number of meanings for the same term or word may be encountered.

This is also the case with the naming of postures. Many of the Sanskrit posture names are indeed standard and will be encountered in all Yoga studios throughout the world, but don't be surprised if a posture introduced by one name in this handbook is called by some other Sanskrit name in another or by your Yoga teacher. Because the teaching tradition in Yoga has been oral rather than written, and is esoteric in nature, this has resulted in some degree of ambiguity in interpretation, as is also the case with many other ancient texts, as experts have interpreted and translated in different ways.

This handbook follows a commonly accepted system of posture names, based on the studies and teachings of a number of Yoga teachers and their varying approaches.

Modern street art from Kathmandu, depicting the ancient Hindu deities and the way in which they rule over the chakras.

Yoga

Yoga is a psychological, physiological and spiritual discipline that has been an integral part of Indian culture for thousands of years. The ancient Yogis developed the system as a means of achieving harmony within themselves and in relation to their environment. They believed that by working with the body and the breath, control over the mind, emotions and general wellbeing could be achieved.

Yoga philosophy was passed down by oral tradition, as it was received by sages through meditation. For this reason, the precise origins of Yoga remain somewhat of a mystery.

The first recorded written mention of Yoga appears in a collection of Indian scriptures called the Vedas, which date back to about 1500BC. However, archaeological finds in the Indus Valley, of intact ceramics depicting figures in Yogic meditation poses, show that Yoga was practised at least 5000 years ago. The practice of Yoga was systematized in approximately the third century BC by a Yogi called Patanjali in his work *The Yoga Sutras*.

Yoga was introduced into the West by an Indian sage called Swami Vivekananda, who demonstrated Yoga postures at a World Fair in Chicago in the 1890s. This generated much interest and laid the grounds for the welcoming of many other Yogis and Swamis from India in the years that followed.

Yoga thrives throughout the world today. Yoga postures have infiltrated today's physical culture in a number of ways: they can be identified in aerobics, stretch and strength routines as well as in warm-ups for dance, sports and gymnastics.

Many of the Yoga postures have been adapted and simplified for the Western body, which may not have grown up steeped in its practice. For example, in the West people are brought up to sit on chairs, whereas in India people are accustomed to sitting cross-legged or squatting. In Indian culture, children are often introduced to Yoga at a very young age, giving them a head start in their levels of flexibility.

In the West, therefore, it takes years of dedicated practice to achieve some of the complex postures, thus necessitating progressive levels in the teaching of Yoga. The tensions of modern life also cause a reduction in flexibility.

If you are new to Yoga, be patient and kind in the treatment of your body. Start at a level relative to your capabilities and limitations. This handbook will guide your steady progress through to a more advanced level over time (read the guide to using this book on page 13).

DIFFERENT SCHOOLS OF YOGA

Most schools adhere to certain basic elements of Yoga, with a slightly different slant on teaching and practice. The four most common schools are Iyengar Yoga, Sivananda Yoga, Ashtanga Yoga and Kundalini Yoga.

Iyengar Yoga was developed by BKS Iyengar, who was born in India in 1918 and still lives there today. This is the most widely recognized form, and much of today's 'Yoga vocabulary' is based on his teachings. His book *Light on Yoga*, published in 1966, has helped spread his teachings worldwide, and has been translated into 18 languages.

Iyengar Yoga is a precise system, concentrating on the physical alignment of postures and often making use of props such as ropes, straps, blocks and chairs to assist the student.

Sivananda Yoga was developed by the medical doctor Swami Sivananda, who was born in South India in 1887. One of his disciples, Swami Vishnu Devananda, introduced Sivananda Yoga to the West in the 1950s, and there are now about 80 Sivananda Yoga centres in the world.

This is a versatile approach, based on 12 key postures, posture variations, the sun salutation, breathing techniques, meditation and chanting. It is a particularly adaptable form of Yoga, from a gentle approach to a more rigorous one.

Ashtanga Yoga, taught by Sri K Pattabhi Jois, is based on an ancient manuscript called the *Yoga Korunta*, rediscovered in the early 20th century. This manuscript contains a system of Hatha Yoga, believed to be the practice intended by Patanjali in the *Yoga Sutras* to integrate the 'eight limbs' of Yoga. The *Yoga Korunta* was deciphered and organized by Pattabhi Jois and his guru Krishnamacharya in the 1930s and is currently taught in many countries. This is an athletic and physically demanding form of Yoga, yet it does allow beginners to follow a progression towards the Primary Series, by working gradually from posture to posture.

Kundalini Yoga is based on the teachings of the Sikh master Yogi Bhajan, who introduced the system to the West in 1969 and founded the 3HO Organization (Healthy, Happy, Holy Organization) in America. This form of Yoga makes use of a breathing technique called 'the fire breath' while executing postures, and focuses on hand and finger gestures, body locks, chanting and meditation. Kundalini Yoga aims to awaken the dormant energy reserve at the base of the spine and raise this energy to the head area.

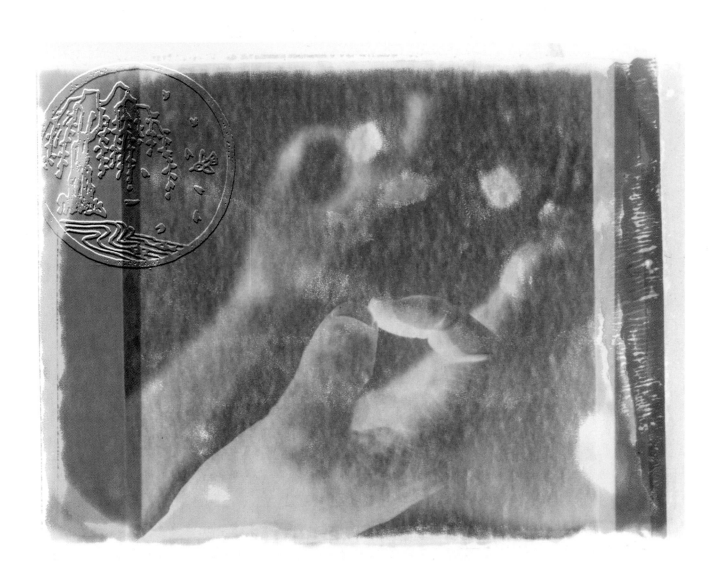

CHAPTER 2

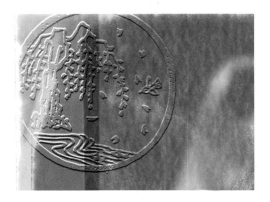

THE SIX BASIC ELEMENTS OF YOGA

The six basic elements of Yoga

The six basic elements of Yoga are posture, breathing, relaxation, meditation, diet and right thinking.

POSTURE

The basic or starting point for all movement is posture, and should therefore be comfortable and stable.

On a physical level, an unhealthy posture can result in the muscles having to carry out some of the work of the bones in maintaining uprightness. This can strain the body and contribute towards chronic back pain or problems such as slipped discs and injuries of the knee, ankle, shoulder or hip.

On a psychological level, the disposition, or psychological and emotional state, is reflected and influenced by the posture. For example, if your shoulders are hunched, your chest collapsed and your head stooped, it could be a sign that you are inwardly 'down'. A chronic deflated posture could indicate deflated sense of self.

A confident person usually holds the head high, with the shoulders open and chest forward or inflated. However, if this posture is extreme, it could indicate an inflated sense of self. A healthy posture, on the other hand, reflects a sense of inner balance and peace.

What is a healthy posture?

A healthy posture is one where only the necessary amount of tension required in the muscles to support the body in uprightness is present – in other words, there is no excess, unnecessary tension. The shoulders are dropped, with the chest open to allow for easy breathing. The arms hang loosely from the shoulders. The feet are well planted on the ground, the knees are not locked and the weight is evenly distributed between both legs and feet.

Such a posture also involves the symmetry of the two sides of the body and is facilitated by muscular balance and the alignment of the skeleton. It includes a lengthening upwards from the waist, so that head and upper body feel poised and light, accompanied by a sense that the legs and feet are well grounded, providing a stable foundation for the body. Breathing is regular and easy, and flows naturally.

The Yoga postures are designed to promote this poised, healthy posture. This is achieved by adopting different positions of the body, each designed to stretch, strengthen, tone and open the body, with a particular focus on the spinal column.

The benefits of this balanced posture are numerous. The body can be used with increased energy, flexibility, ease and awareness, and the internal workings of the body function optimally. The life force flows more freely throughout the body, increasing the sense of vitality. Breathing also becomes easier and more free. The skeletal structure is grounded and brought into better alignment, while the nervous system perceives stability and allows the muscles to release unnecessary tension.

Finally, a healthy posture results in greater ease and satisfaction in the way we do the Yoga postures, and it speeds up the rate at which we improve. Working to improve posture also influences the way we feel about ourselves and therefore the way in which we relate to others.

How to achieve a healthy posture

When you are standing or sitting, try to lengthen your spine (from the tailbone to the crown) without straining – imagine that you are being suspended from the sky by an invisible string.

A. Stand with your legs together or slightly apart, and aim to position your eyes, ears, shoulders, hips, knees and ankles parallel to the ground.

B. From a side view, you should be able to draw a straight line downward from the crown of your head, in front of your ear, through the centre of your shoulder, the centre of your hip, behind the kneecap and through or just in front of your anklebone. Be sure to distribute your weight evenly between both legs and try not to lock your knees.

Extend the back of your neck while holding your chin parallel to the ground; you may prefer to drop your chin slightly. This encourages a lengthening of the upper portion of the spine, with a balanced sense of a strong back and a soft front.

C. The weight under your feet should be evenly distributed under three points of each foot: under the big toe's metatarsal, the little toe's metatarsal and the heel. Press your abdomen lightly against your spine, to encourage extension and length in the spine from the lower back.

D&E. The same techniques apply when you are sitting, from the head to the hips. To help keep your back straight, you may need to sit on a cushion or on your haunches, so that your hips are slightly raised above your knees.

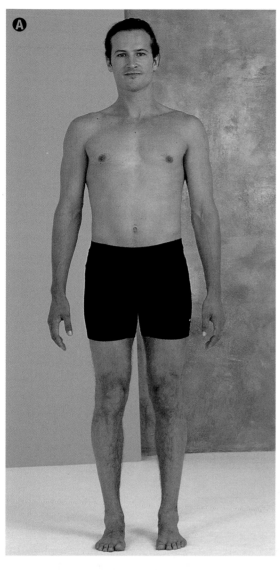

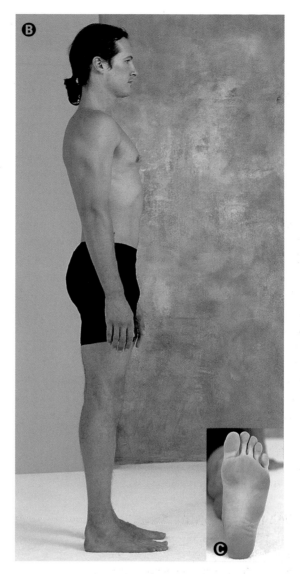

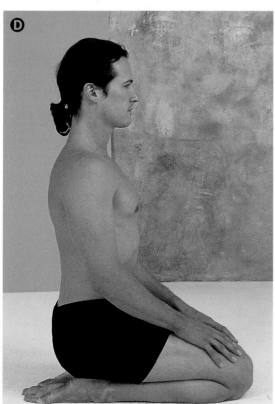

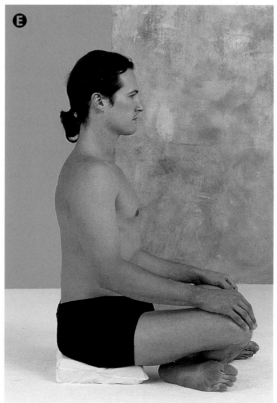

Breathing

Breathing, the ever-alternating movement between inhalation and exhalation, is considered to be the most important of all human functions. We are able to exist for several days without eating and fewer days without drinking, but only minutes without breathing.

We are not only dependent upon breathing for life, but our sense of vitality is linked directly to our breathing habits and patterns. Yet with poor posture, contracted chests and stooped shoulders, our breathing is often quick and shallow. Yoga is perhaps the only system of exercise that focuses extensively on breathing as an intrinsic part of practice. Conscious and controlled breathing serves as an accompaniment to the physical postures, as well as a practice in its own right. The breath is found to assist flow of movement, as well as to help the mind focus on the present moment.

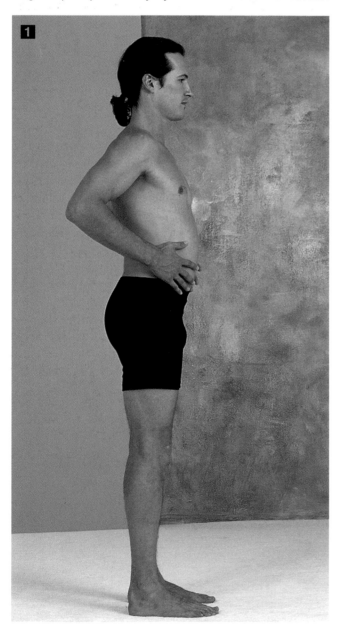

Breathing and life force

The Sanskrit word Pranayama refers to the breathing practices of Yoga. 'Prana' means 'energy' or 'life force' and 'yama' means 'to lengthen'. The main aim of Pranayama, then, as the name implies, is to bring about increased vitality and improve the quality of our lives and health, through lengthening the breath and training in the art of breathing more deeply and fully.

In Yoga, breathing is both a physical act as well as a process of receiving that vital energy or life force from the universe. Prana is the life force that animates all forms of life in the universe; it permeates every cell in the human body and is the force behind the renewal and revitalizing of every cell. Thus health and vitality are dependent upon the amount of prana that infuses the body.

One way in which prana is absorbed into the body is through the breath. Breathing more fully and efficiently will therefore increase the amount of prana in the body, nourishing the tissues, the bloodstream and the nerves and increasing the general sense of vitality.

This does not imply, though, that deeper breathing is always better, as it is possible to hyperventilate from taking in too much breath too quickly. What is referred to here is learning to become aware of and to gain conscious control over the breath as much as possible.

Proper breathing and physical health

Controlled, deep breathing helps to calm the nervous system and relax the body and mind. This can be helpful in countering insomnia or poor-quality sleep.

Breathing oxygenates the brain and clears the mind. At the same time it oxygenates the tissues and the cells of the bloodstream and nerves, keeping them nourished. It helps to improve blood circulation, as well as the functioning of the immune system, while deep breathing can be used effectively to alleviate and treat asthma and bronchitis.

1. The proper use of the diaphragm in deep breathing massages the abdominal organs on inhalation, as it moves downward to increase the lung capacity. This action aids the digestion process.
2. On exhalation, the diaphragm gently massages the heart. The strong pumping action of the diaphragm influences the flow of fluids throughout the lymphatic system, so the more the diaphragm is exercised, the greater the detoxification effect. When the emphasis of deep breathing is on the inhalation, it helps to counter low blood pressure. When the emphasis is on lengthening the exhalation, this helps to counter high blood pressure.

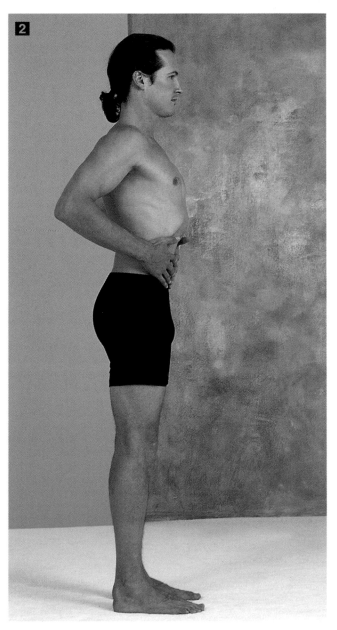

Breathing and the emotions

Proper breathing is intrinsically linked with the emotions and the state of mind. For example, when we are frightened, we gasp inwards and hold our breath. When we are tired or bored, our breathing is long and drawn out – we yawn. Breathing becomes irregular and choppy with anger or sorrow, while with tension, worry or anxiety, the breath becomes shallow and either slow or hurried.

Because the breath and the emotions are interdependent, it is possible to reduce the effects of emotional turbulence by bringing the breath under control. At any point we are able to choose to breathe more evenly, calmly and deeply. You'll soon discover that it is not possible to feel anxious when breathing in a calm, controlled manner. On the other hand, of course, it is not possible to feel calm when breathing is jerky, hurried and uneven.

How to breathe properly

All breathing in Yoga (unless otherwise specified) is through the nose. The nose contains little hairs that filter, warm and moisten the air before it enters the lungs; through the mouth the air with all its pollutants is passed, unfiltered, directly into the lungs.

Breathing, in most Yoga postures, begins from a healthy posture. To allow maximum exercising of the diaphragm, the lower abdomen is held slightly contracted (pressed lightly towards the spine) and breathing is into the ribcage and upper abdominal area, between the navel and the ribcage.

1. On inhalation, expand the upper abdomen and ribcage, taking care to breathe into the front and the back of the ribcage.
2. On exhalation, relax the ribcage and lower abdomen to allow air to flow out, and activate the abdominal muscles towards the end of the exhalation to help expel as much air as possible. (Contraction of the abdominal muscles causes the diaphragm to press upwards and compress the lungs, helping the lungs to empty fully.)

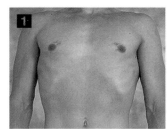
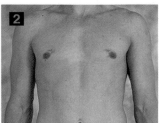

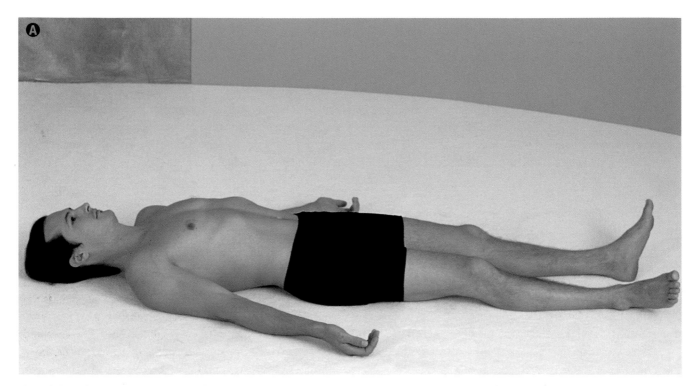

RELAXATION

Relaxation allows the body time to replenish its energy reserves in preparation for the next activity or another day. It is a natural counterpart to the state of tension.

While a certain amount of tension is necessary in order to maintain the uprightness of the body, a certain amount of relaxation is also necessary in order to bring flow to our movement and functioning.

In this context, relaxation is the ability to let go completely, while lying down or sitting still. This will assist you to move through life with reduced levels of unnecessary tension and attain mental focus and the ability to concentrate.

In Yoga, relaxation exercises allow the body to absorb and integrate the energy released through the various postures. This allows the practitioner to gain the full benefit from each posture or series of postures.

Relaxation also allows time for the blood to circulate throughout the body, after holding Yoga postures which concentrate the blood in specific areas of the body.

The effects of tension

Most people have experienced accumulated muscular tension in response to stress, where muscles are unable to return to a balanced, resting state. The result is that too much effort is used to carry out any action, however simple. These tensions become a habit, and that's how we carry ourselves every day.

The overall effects of such tension may include reduced energy levels, reduced flexibility, restriction to the free flow of breath and a reduction of the efficiency of any activity. Tension also results in increased vulnerability to injury, sickness, fatigue or sleep problems.

How Yoga can help

The process of letting go of muscular tension is often gradual, especially when the tension has been accumulated over many years. It also takes a while to learn how to maintain a relaxed and balanced state during stressful situations.

The practice of Yoga takes this into account and uses relaxation techniques as an integral part of the practice. The postures, breathing and mental focus exercises have a calming

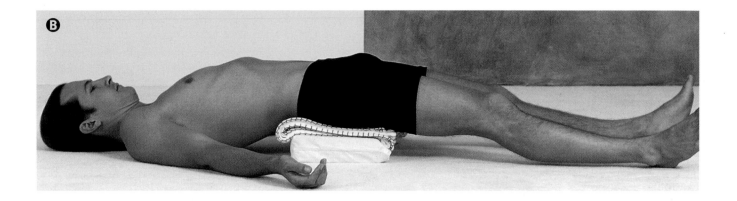

and soothing effect on the mind and body, helping to activate the parasympathetic (calming) nervous system. There are also specific relaxation exercises for letting go of muscular tension. These exercises are incorporated before, during and after the Yoga session in order to encourage a relaxed, easy and unforced approach to the practice of Yoga (A, B & C). This calmness filters naturally into the Yoga practitioner's everyday life.

The relaxed mind

It takes just as much – if not more – conscious effort to relax and silence the mind and release mental tension as it takes to relax muscular tension in the body. Thus many practitioners believe that the relaxation postures are the most difficult Yoga postures to truly master.

Mental relaxation is not to be confused with mental sluggishness. Allowing yourself time to relax your mind has the same revitalizing effect as allowing yourself time to relax your body. The result is clarity of thought, mental calmness and enhanced concentration; a sluggish mind is marked by a decrease in these capacities.

Concentrating on and deepening the breath is one effective way of calming the mind. It brings the attention of the mind into the present moment, leaving behind the hopes and fears belonging to the past or the future.

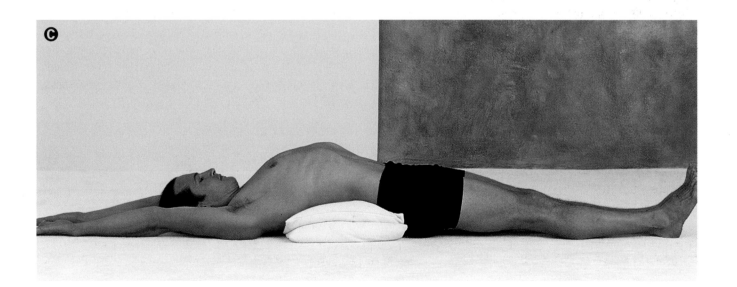

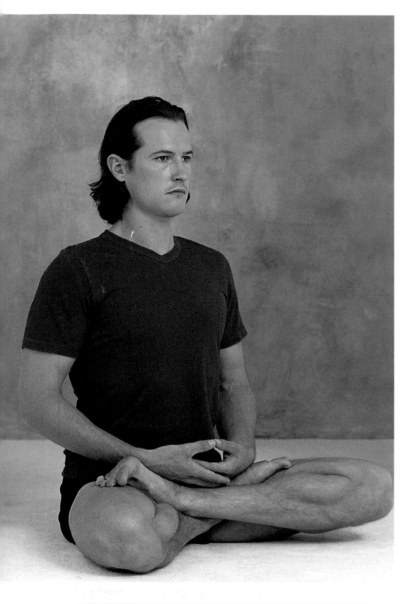

MEDITATION

A basic premise in Yoga is that a healthy state of awareness involves the ability to focus and maintain the attention on the present moment. Meditation is one Yogic method of achieving this focus.

Meditation generally refers to the act of contemplation or reflection on the self, on the nature of the mind or on something greater than the self, whether that is viewed as God, universal consciousness or any chosen symbol of divinity. Meditation is not something that is learned – it is a state that arises naturally out of regular practice of mental focus or concentration.

Although meditation is often associated with certain religious paths or rituals, in this book the term is used to describe an ancient practice used to quieten the mind and work towards greater self-knowledge and self-mastery. Also, the act of meditation as presented here does not promote any particular religion.

The benefits of meditation

Meditation cultivates a state of contentment and serenity. It induces brain-wave states of mental relaxation and calmness and has been found to regulate blood pressure. It also activates the parasympathetic nervous system, which exerts a calming influence and allows the muscles of the body to let go of unnecessary tension, and helps to regulate breathing patterns. When practised daily, for anything from five minutes to one or more hours, meditation is an effective tool for coping with or rising above the challenges and potentially stressful situations that life may present.

On a spiritual dimension, concentration of the attention and the resultant quieting of the mind's chatter and activity leads to true meditation, which involves a withdrawal of the senses so that one is not distracted. The ultimate aim of meditation is the triggering of a state of bliss and a super-conscious state, with its heightened awareness, enlightenment or intuitive realization of the nature of the self.

The difference between relaxation and meditation

Relaxation does not necessarily require alertness or any particular focus of attention. It is a state close to sleep, and if maintained would lead to sleep.

Meditation, on the other hand, involves the training of a heightened state of awareness and alertness through

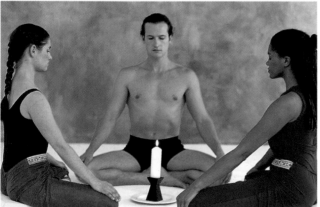

concentrating the attention on the present moment (often focusing on a chosen object, image, word, phrase or emotion). It is a state of being awake and alert, yet calm and focused.

Both relaxation and meditation in Yoga offer valuable skills for finding and maintaining a state of calmness, which can help when confronted with stressful situations.

To gain the maximum benefit from Yoga, it is important to practise both Hatha Yoga and meditation. Traditionally, Hatha Yoga is seen as a preparation for better meditation, as the postures, breathing and relaxation practices relieve the body of tensions and tone the nervous system, which result in reduced restlessness when sitting still to meditate. The postures and breathing also begin the process of focusing the mind and learning to maintain this focus in the present moment, which is the ultimate goal of meditation.

Regular meditation practice, in turn, is also helpful to the practice of Hatha Yoga, as meditation further tones the nervous system, thus cultivating a state of calmness and serenity. Meditation helps to identify areas of tension that may be hindering the practice of postures and it helps to gain greater control over the mind's chatter that may distract the practice of Yoga and the ability to truly relax.

Helpful pointers on meditation practice

- Do Yoga, go for a walk or do some activity before meditating. This helps to reduce restlessness.
- It may help to do about five minutes of Pranayama before meditating, as this helps to calm and settle the mind and body.
- Try to meditate at the same time each day. This will help the mind expect a period of silence at that time. Meditation in the morning helps to prepare the mind for the day, and at night it helps to rid the body of tensions and the mind of mental activity before sleep.
- Meditate in the same place each day, if possible.
- Start with a shorter period of meditation, such as five or 10 minutes, in order to gradually build up your silence-stamina.
- Try to lengthen this time progressively (perhaps setting monthly goals, building up from five to 10 or 20 minutes). Work towards sitting for more or less 45 minutes every day, or at least three times a week.
- When sitting, do a mental body check to relax each part of your body from head to toe. Remember to check your facial muscles, as they often hold tension.
- Focus the mind and/or the eyes in a relaxed manner, on the subject or object of choice.

- Overleaf, three meditation techniques are presented, all aimed at assisting the mind to focus on the present moment. If you know of any other technique, perhaps learned in a Yoga class, feel free to apply the technique that you find most helpful.
- If the mind wanders and thoughts and emotions come up (as they will), allow them to pass through your mind (and body) and then let them go by bringing the attention back to the chosen subject or object. This may happen repeatedly while meditating. The idea is to keep returning to the focus of attention without becoming angry. In time, it will become easier to let thoughts pass without being drawn into or distracted by them.
- It is also helpful to label any thoughts that arise as 'thinking', so that all thoughts are made equal. This helps to bring awareness to the process of thinking as well as to the spaces between thoughts. It is these spaces that meditation aims to lengthen.
- If you find you get drowsy, it could be for a number of reasons. Question whether you have had enough sleep the night before. Drowsiness could also be mistaken for the welcome release of tension in the body, and it could also be understood as an unconscious resistance to awareness. Either way, try not to give in to such drowsiness, as in time your concentration will improve and your nervous system will get used to periods of stillness.

Sitting positions for meditation

For each of the sitting positions, you can limber up your hip and knee joints by using Baddha Konasana (p68).

Sit on a cushion or folded blanket, so that your hips are slightly raised above the level of your knees. This helps to sit upright more comfortably. (The only exception is the Full Lotus position, suitable for advanced practitioners, which may not require raised hips for stability.)

You may also want to sit on a soft surface, like a carpet, mat or blanket, so that your knees are comfortable on the ground.

Sit with your spine extending upwards with ease, all the way up through the back of your neck and head. Slightly press the lower abdomen towards the spine, to assist in keeping the lower back straight.

Breathe into the upper torso by allowing mainly the ribcage and the upper abdomen (between the navel and the ribcage) to expand. Be aware of breathing into the back and the front of the ribcage.

Sukhasana (also known as Muktasana)

1. Sukhasana means a comfortable and steady sitting position, so all you need do is sit with your legs crossed comfortably. Adapt this position to suit your needs (for example, if you have a knee injury, sit with one leg straight).

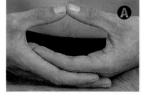 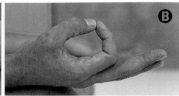

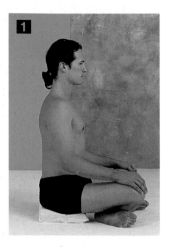

Siddhasana

2. Start in Sukhasana and take hold of one ankle or foot and place it on top of the other, ideally with the outer edge of the raised foot pressing into the opposite groin. It can be simplified by placing the ankle onto the opposite thigh or by placing one ankle or calf on top of the other. This is a preparation for Padmasana. Swap legs if you use this position regularly, to develop flexibility evenly in both legs and hips.

Padmasana (the Full Lotus)

1. Start in Sukhasana.
2. Move into Siddhasana.
3. Lift the other leg, pressing the outer edge of the foot into the opposite groin. Take hold of your feet and ease them further into the groin area, aiming for a balanced, symmetrical position.

Hand positions

The hand positions are designed to help centre the energy in your body by creating a closed circuit for the energy to circulate.

Place your hands on your knees or thighs, so that your elbows rest at your sides and your shoulders are relaxed.

Choose one of the following hand positions: rest your right hand in your left (A); rest both hands on your thighs or knees, with palms facing down; or assume the Chin Mudra position, with both hands on the thighs or knees, palms facing up and the tips of the forefinger and thumb touching (B).

MEDITATION TECHNIQUES

Focus on the breath

Focus your attention on your breath by simply watching your breath, without changing it in any way.

Breathing is through the nose, with the attention more on the out-breath (and a lengthening of the out-breath) than on the in-breath.

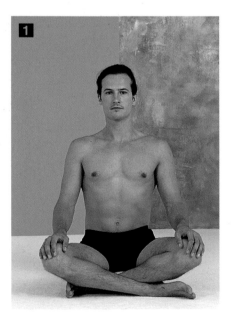 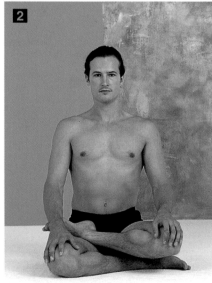 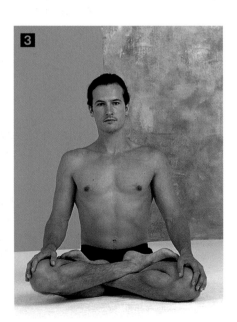

Sense a letting go of tensions, thoughts and emotions with each out-breath, particularly at the end of the out-breath, as you await the next in-breath.

This technique can be practised with eyes open or closed. If the eyes are open, rest your eyes on a chosen point of focus, on the ground a few feet away from your body, or at eye level on, for example, a candle flame. If your eyes are closed, focus your attention solely on the breath.

This technique is particularly effective for calming the emotions and clearing the mind by relieving mental tension arising from anxiety and confusion.

Focus on an object

Place a lit candle (or any object) either at eye level in front of you (on a low table) or on the floor a few feet away from you, so that when your spine is lengthened, your eyes are gently downcast, focusing neither too close nor too far from your body. Aim to keep your attention on the flame as you gaze at the candle. If your mind wanders, return your attention to the candle flame as soon as you notice.

If you wish, after you have been gazing at the candle for a few minutes, close your eyes and visualize the candle flame at the centre point between your eyebrows. Hold this vision until you return your gaze to the flame. You can alternate the open and closed eyes, holding each for no less than a minute.

This candle-gazing technique helps increase the concentration span. It is also a fun way to meditate with the whole family, as the whole family can sit together in a circle and focus on the same candle in the centre.

This exercise can be practiced with any other object, too, such as a flower, or a stone. The object should be as simple as possible, so that the mind is not distracted by, for example, examining intricate decoration on an ornament.

Repetition of the Ohm sound

Add to the focused breath meditation the repetition of the 'Ohm' sound, once on inhalation and once on exhalation. Repeat the sound silently in your mind or say it out loud.

Sacred sounds, such as the universal Ohm sound (written

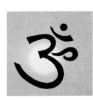

in Sanskrit at left), serve as an effective means of calming and clearing the mind and cultivating an experience of peace and contentment.

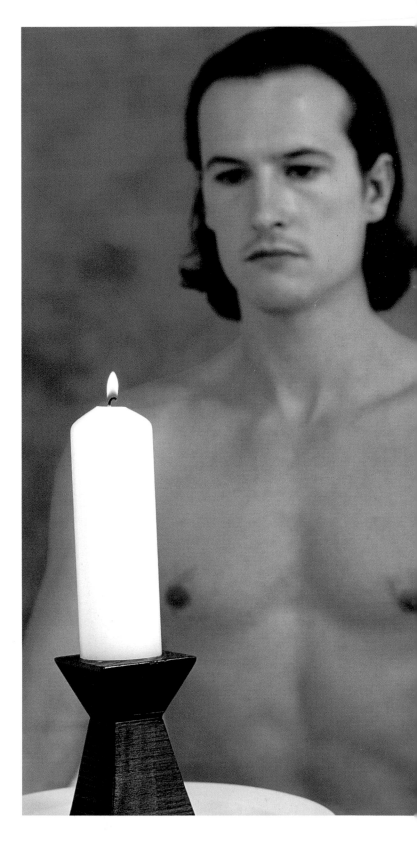

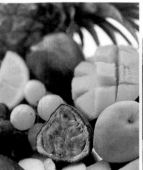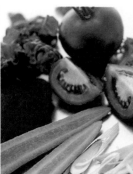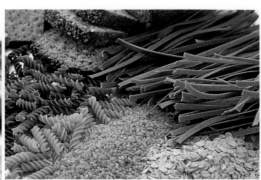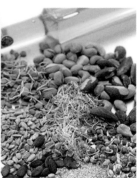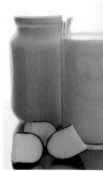

DIET

Within the Yoga philosophy, food is believed to have both physiological and psychological effects. Certain kinds of foods influence the body and mind in ways that are either beneficial or detrimental to health.

Rajasic foods

These foods are stimulating and include caffeine-containing products, refined sugar, onion, garlic, chilli and anything that is strongly spiced or flavoured or extremely bitter, sour, salty, pungent or sweet. When consumed in excess, Rajasic foods over-stimulate the endocrine and nervous system and agitate the mind, therefore getting in the way of Yoga and the state of calmness and contentment.

Tamasic foods

These foods are depressing, rob us of energy and poison the system. Tamasic foods include stale, tasteless, putrefied or overripe foods, foods that are not fresh, such as tinned, frozen, processed or preserved products, meat and alcohol.

Sattvic foods

These foods are pure and life-giving, such as fresh fruits and vegetables, nuts, seeds, beans, wholegrains, dairy and honey.

General guidelines for a healthy diet

A healthy, Sattvic diet is a lacto-vegetarian diet, with fruits, vegetables, nuts, seeds, grains, legumes/beans as well as dairy products, and very little Rajasic and Tamasic foods.

While it may be difficult to change a lifetime of eating habits, challenge yourself to try these principles for a few months to experience the benefits.

If you make the decision to reduce your meat intake or stop altogether, it will be necessary to allow the body enough time to adjust to the new diet.

Perhaps the most important thing is to eat foods as close as possible to their natural state, as food is then at its freshest and most nourishing, and most infused with life force (prana). Such foods not only are easy to digest, but can also improve sluggish digestion and help to promote a healthy colon.

- Eat plenty of fruits, vegetables and sprouted beans/legumes.
- Choose fresh produce over frozen, processed, tinned or pre-prepared produce.
- Eat nuts and seeds in moderation – they are valuable sources of essential fatty acids and protein.
- Choose wholegrain breads and pasta wherever possible.
- Choose yoghurt with live cultures.
- Use honey instead of sugar, and substitute dates, dried fruits or products sweetened with fructose for sweets. Where you can, use carob instead of chocolate.
- Eat a variety of foods.
- Avoid artificially preserved, coloured or flavoured products.
- Avoid oily, fried foods.
- Try to cut down on red meat and chicken and focus on fish, which is lighter and easier to digest. If you wish to eat chicken and eggs, opt for the free-range variety.
- Whatever you choose to eat, eat slowly and chew your food well. Digestion starts in the mouth with the mixing of food with saliva. The stomach can tolerate almost anything if chewed thoroughly.
- Eat in moderation – in other words, eat until you are satisfied and not overly full. A healthy way to think of this is to fill two-thirds of the stomach's capacity, allowing one-third to remain empty. In this way, the stomach is able to process food optimally.
- Allow sufficient time between meals for the stomach to empty and an appetite to develop.
- Aim to cut out smoking, alcohol, caffeine and any other stimulants or depressants you use out of habit. These substances can hinder your progress in Yoga as well as your health in general.

Note: Consult your health practitioner when embarking on a major dietary change as your body may start to detoxify and display symptoms that, although temporary, may be alleviated through herbal or medical assistance.

Fasting

People fast for many different reasons, such as for health, religious reasons or as a mental discipline.

From a health perspective, going without solid foods for a day or so is like a tonic for the system. It gives the digestive system a break, thus allowing more energy to be concentrated on the cleansing, detoxifying functions of the vital organs.

Advanced Yoga practitioners can go without solid foods for extended periods of time, but the average person should fast only in moderation. Select one day a week or month where you take in only fruits and liquids, or only liquids.

As a mental discipline, fasting helps to overcome the feeling of being controlled by the senses. It helps to gain control over the cravings and desires for food that often control us.

Note: Any extended fast should be embarked upon only under supervision and with the consent of your health practitioner, as detoxification symptoms can become overwhelming.

A LIFE OF RIGHT ACTION

To gain the most out of Yoga, a certain awareness and caring needs to filter through into all aspects of life. Yoga is concerned with the health and vitality of body, mind and spirit and all that can bring about that health. How we think, speak and act are all important, and can either hold us back or accelerate our progress in Yoga.

We should also aim to extend our caring towards others, by not harming any living creature through thought, word or action. Through our own personal progress and radiance that results from our caring, we not only can improve the quality of our own lives but also influence the lives of all who we encounter.

Ethical disciplines (Yama)

In his *Yoga Sutras*, Patanjali points out certain fundamental ethical disciplines that form the basis of Yoga and are the guidelines for moral behaviour in society.

One such discipline is non-violence (Ahimsa), which includes a non-violent attitude towards oneself, others and life.

We live in a world where violence, intimidation and war are among the more common methods of affecting change. This violence originates in thought (in thinking a negative thought about another person or wishing bad upon another), which can be expressed as words and translated into action. Thus the place to start affecting change is in the mind and attitude of the individual.

This attitude of violence also manifests on a personal level, towards the self, in habits such as self-deprecation and criticism. If you treat yourself in this way, you are likely to treat others in this way too. So begin by cultivating a nurturing, caring, gentle and kind attitude towards yourself. Even an intention in this direction will begin the process of identifying habits of thought, speech and action, which will become noticeable and thus available for change.

This ethical discipline of non-violence also influences the Yogic dietary philosophy as a reason for refraining from eating meat or limiting one's intake of meat. It is an act of non-violence and respect towards the animal kingdom.

Truthfulness (Satya), like non-violence, begins with the self. To what extent are you truthful with yourself about your behaviour, interactions and achievements? The more people strive for truthfulness in their lives, the faster such an attitude will spread.

The other ethical disciplines are non-stealing (Asteya), chastity (Brahmacarya – this may be interpreted as controlling the sexual urge and, if one chooses to be sexually active, then not to abuse it or become a slave to it) and non-covetousness (Aparigraha – being satisfied with what you have and not hoarding things for which you no longer have a need).

Personal practices or disciplines (Niyama)

These disciplines help to maintain the ethical disciplines.

- Cleanliness of the mind and body (Saucha) – internal and external hygiene
- Contentment (Santosa) – if you are not content within your own mind and being, it is far more difficult to be caring and giving to yourself or to anyone else
- Austerity (Tapas) – a burning desire to better yourself and under all circumstances to strive towards the union between the individual and the Divine
- Study of the scriptures (Svadhyaya) – studying ancient and modern texts and commentaries in order to educate yourself
- Surrender or dedication to the Divine (Isvara Pranidhana) – having faith in the Divine as a general guiding motivation.

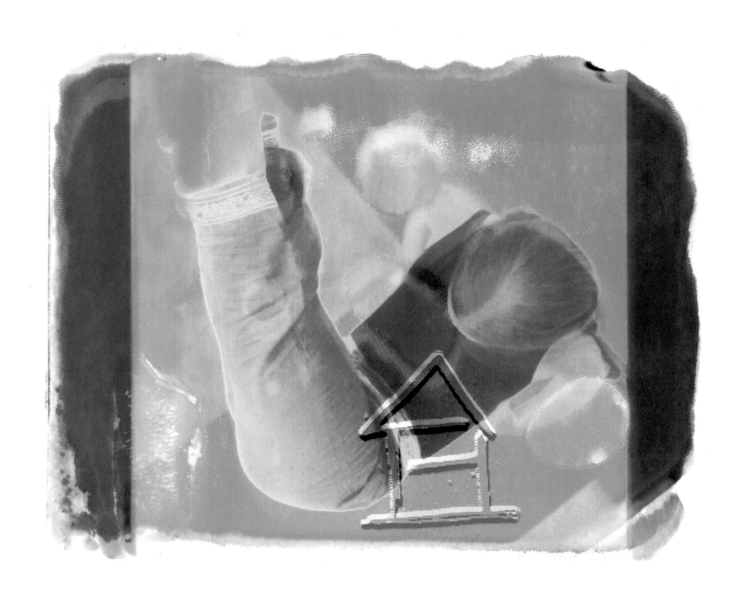

CHAPTER 3

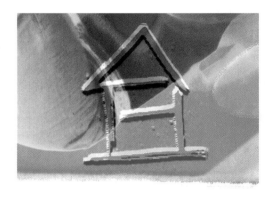

PRACTISING YOGA AT HOME

Practising Yoga at home

Even if you intend practising much of your Yoga at home, it is a good idea to join a local Yoga class in addition to learning Yoga from this handbook.

New postures should first be tried out under a teacher's supervision, as a teacher provides valuable supervision in checking the correct alignment of the body in postures. On your own, you are not always able to feel when your alignment is correct, and a position may feel upright or symmetrical when in fact it is not. This can lead to strain or injury.

A teacher will demonstrate how to ease your body into and out of a posture, as well as remind you how to breathe while holding a posture (A & B). Having the posture demonstrated in front of you also helps for clarification.

Apart from the fact that a class atmosphere can be fun and encouraging, a Yoga teacher will point out where you may be limiting yourself and offer ways to help you achieve the desired posture.

Nevertheless, there are many advantages to being able to practise Yoga at home. For example, you can choose the time of day that suits your schedule – this is particularly useful if you have children or a heavy work schedule. You are also able to choose the length of session, and can focus on a certain posture or group of postures. This is also useful for practising a posture that you may have struggled with in a class or that you find particularly challenging.

On your own, you can take all the time you want, without having to work at the pace of others. And you will improve your flexibility and strength more quickly if you practise at home as well as attending a class.

telephone. Make sure that the room temperature is moderate to warm, not too hot or cold. Avoid practising in direct sunlight or if you have just returned inside from spending time in the hot sun.

The surface on which you practise must be firm and level. If it is carpeted, rather work on a large bath towel, rug or folded blanket. On a wooden floor or any other smooth surface, use a non-slip mat (C) – if you can't find one through your local Yoga centre, use a camping mat.

If you wish to practise outside, choose a grassy patch of garden or a sandy beach. If your garden has no lawn, cover the surface with a sponge mat, layered blanket, or towels to create a soft surface area (D). Once again, make sure that the area is free from disturbances.

Select comfortable, loose-fitting or elasticized clothing to allow complete freedom of movement and avoid any restricting of breathing or circulation.

Although your feet should be bare, if it is really cold you can wear a pair of socks until you warm up. Remove your jewellery where practical.

Do not eat directly before practice, and allow three to four hours after a heavy meal and one to two hours after a light snack.

Empty the bladder and bowels if possible before practice (some of the postures will assist bowel movement, so this is not an essential before getting started).

Try to shower or bath before practice, or sponge down or splash your face, arms, hands and feet to freshen up. Postures will come easier after a warm bath, which will assist your practice.

Preparation for Yoga at home

Yoga can be practised inside or outside the home, and you will probably find that your home is already a fully equipped Yoga gymnasium. The few items you may need to buy should see you through many rewarding years of practice.

You will need to practise in a clear, open space, large enough to stretch your limbs while standing and lying down. Move the furniture if necessary. The area should be clean and quiet. If possible, turn on the answering machine or unplug the

Helpful props

- Two to four cushions
- A long strap (up to 2m, 6ft long) or a belt
- A block (or a pile of books, depending on their sizes)
- A blanket to keep warm during relaxation (if necessary) and to fold to provide a soft surface
- A chair
- A full-length mirror (optional) to assist you in checking your alignment in postures

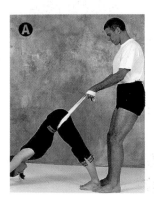
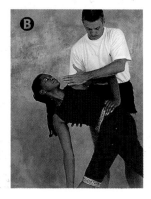
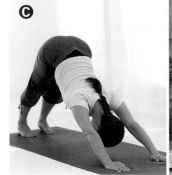
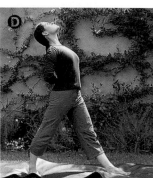

How often to practise

It would be ideal to practise Yoga every day, although particularly in the beginning this is not always possible. Remember that it is important to enjoy your practice, so it should not be enforced as a strict and harsh discipline. Be gentle with yourself and pay attention to how you are feeling each day, adjusting your Yoga practice accordingly.

When to practise

Try to set aside the same time each day, as consistency helps to encourage discipline and offers the most rewards. So choose a time when you know you will not be rushed or disturbed. The best times to practise are in the early morning or early evening.

In the morning, your mind is fresh, alert and more determined, although your muscles may be a little stiff. Thus a morning practice is particularly good for loosening up stiff muscles and preparing your mind and body for the day.

In the evening, your body moves with greater ease and is more flexible, but your mind may be tired. An evening practice is particularly good for unwinding and releasing the stress and tension of the day.

Nevertheless, whatever the time of day, Yoga practice will refresh and calm your body and mind. Experiment to decide which you prefer, or which fits better into your schedule or the season (it may be easier to rise early in summer).

You may also need to make some adjustments to your practice, depending on the season – the cooling breath (Sithali), for example, is designed for practise in hot weather. The instructions accompanying the techniques will guide you. You may also find that in cold weather your body needs a longer warm-up. So listen to your body with compassion and kindness and you will find out quickly which postures, practices and times of day suit you. This will help you to gain the most out of your practice.

The length of each practice

A session can last anything from 10 minutes to two hours. It is important to allow time for postures and relaxation, so if you only have time for a short session, choose fewer postures. Never rush your practice.

To gain maximum benefit, set aside 60–90 minutes. This will allow time for postures, breathing practice, relaxation and meditation (for example: 45 minutes postures, with rest poses in between; 5–10 minutes breathing practice; 5–10 minutes relaxation; and anything from 5–30 minutes meditation. Naturally you can juggle your time as you please, allowing more time for postures in a 90-minute practice.) When starting out you may find that you prefer a shorter practice, this is perfectly acceptable. Gradually you will get used to the practice and work your way to a longer session.

Working with a partner or alone

Working with a partner is a fun and helpful variation in your practice. Partners can assist by checking posture and alignment in the various positions, as well as check for undue strain, for example, in the face, while holding a posture, or simply remind each other to breathe. They also can provide support for each other in attempting new or tricky postures or can gently assist in certain stretches.

It also is safer to work with someone who is more experienced than you are, who is familiar with the postures and can help with their execution. And, of course, if anything goes wrong, your partner can help.

If you are working alone, perhaps ask someone to read the instructions to you in the beginning, to allow you to concentrate on the posture or relaxation practice. Rather try out the beginner's postures before attempting more difficult versions. Only if you can comfortably execute these should you move on to more advanced versions. Be cautious in your practice to prevent injury.

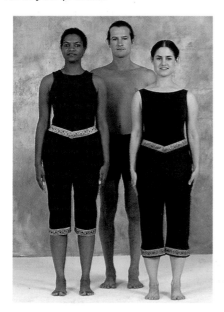

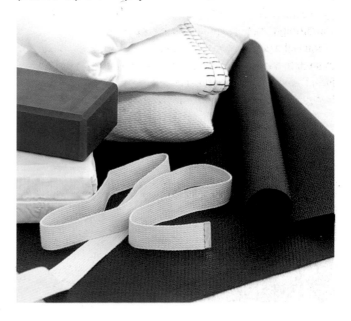

It may be useful to work with a full-length mirror, particularly if you're a beginner, to check your alignment. Try to join a Yoga class that will safely introduce you to the postures and check your execution of them, before attempting practice at home.

In the beginning, keep your eyes open when executing the postures, as this helps your sense of balance. When you are more advanced, you may wish to close your eyes in order to keep your mind focused on your breath and the co-ordination of your breath with movement.

If you are working in a group, you may wish to close your eyes so that you don't compare yourself critically with others. This helps to encourage an introspective and personal approach to your practice. With standing postures and balances you should keep your eyes open.

GENERAL SAFETY PRECAUTIONS

General safety precautions are outlined for each posture and appear on the same pages as the respective postures. Nevertheless, there are some practical tips that apply to the general practice of Yoga, and are important in order to avoid injury:

- Read all the instructions and cautions carefully, or have them read to you.
- Check that your practice area is clear of any sharp objects, balls, objects with wheels or anything that you may be able to stand or slip on or knock over.
- Check that the surface on which you are practising is not slippery, so that you will not have to support your balance with muscles that are not directly involved in the posture (these muscles could be strained). Invest in a rubber Yoga mat if you do not have a non-slip surface plan.
- Be gentle with yourself and never work into pain. If you push yourself too hard, you can strain or sprain a muscle or ligament. Check that you can breathe easily and work within your constructive and realistic limits.
- Never attempt a more difficult version of a posture until you can comfortably execute the simpler version, holding it for at least 30 seconds or eight deep breaths.
- Try to attempt postures for the first time under the supervision of a teacher or someone who is more experienced than you.
- If you are practising alone, make sure that there is a telephone nearby in case you need to call for help.

- If you are tired, Yoga can be revitalizing, but if you are struggling to concentrate, rather rest for a while or do a simple session. Lack of concentration can make you more prone to injury.
- If you know that you have a chronic medical condition such as asthma, diabetes or heart disease, keep your medication with you and preferably practise with a partner for extra safety.

After the session – relaxation outside of the Yoga class

Yoga is a philosophy that can be included in every aspect of your life. You shouldn't treat yourself with gentle care and nurturing only while you're practising Yoga.

If you take note of some of these suggestions, you will allow this attitude to pervade your entire life, to help you maintain a state of health, serenity and mental clarity.

Take time out

At least once a week, try to spend time outdoors, walking in the mountains, in a forest, in a botanical garden or along a beach. Take short breaks outdoors every day, even it is 10 minutes during lunch or tea break.

You could also take 'time out' indoors practising a few full, deep breaths, doing eye exercises or stretching your arms, neck and shoulders, as described in Chapter 4. This offers quick and effective tension relief at any time of day, even if you can spare only 5–10 minutes at your desk.

Another suggestion is to take 10 or more deep breaths when you feel tension building up. You could also close your eyes or allow your eyes to rest on an object in the room, such as a plant. This offers relief after spending long stretches in front of a computer, and you can then return to your work with refreshed focus and renewed concentration.

Develop a hobby

A hobby offers an opportunity for you to do something just for yourself, without having to meet deadlines or accumulate stress in the process.

If your work has grown out of a hobby, find a new hobby, so that you are able to take a break from your regular routine.

Massage therapy

At least once a month, treat yourself to a massage, which will help to release muscular tension.

Massage can also help increase your mobility and encourage flow of movement, which is often restricted by tense holding patterns in the muscles and ligaments. Thus regular massage therapy will complement your practice.

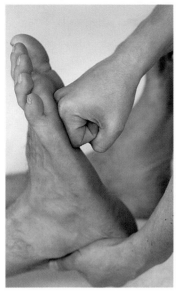
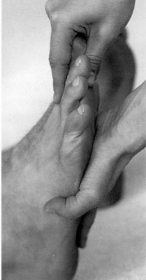

Some massage techniques are gentle, while others involve deeper tissue massage. Try different techniques (such as aromatherapy, Swedish massage, reflexology and Shiatsu) to find one (or more) that works for you.

A massage will also often bring to your awareness areas where you hold tension. With this awareness, you can choose Yoga postures that work on these respective areas, as a means of keeping them in check on a regular basis.

The importance of sleep

Too little sleep is a major contributor to fatigue of the body and mind, and it also results in a general lack of energy for carrying out the tasks of daily living.

A common cause of sleeping problems is the inability to relax or let go of muscular tension. Another possible cause is the inability to quiet the chatter or 'noise' of the mind at the end of the day. Yoga can help you relax more fully and work to still the restless mind, thus improving the quality of your sleep.

DEVISING A YOGA SESSION

It is important to learn to respect and listen to the natural intelligence of your body.

After doing a session of postures you should feel serene, energized and light. If you feel drained and exhausted, then you have probably overdone it. Be gentle with yourself, as pushing too hard can do more harm than good. Harnessing this, together with a knowledge of the cautions and general rules for safe applying Yoga practice, will set you well on your way to devising fun, varied and beneficial Yoga sessions that are suited to your individual needs.

Dynamic versus static postures

To execute a posture dynamically means to move in and out of a posture repeatedly, while co-ordinating breath with movement.

A static posture is one in which the position is held for some period. of time, counted in breaths (such as for three to eight breaths). Nevertheless, it is important to remember that static postures are actively held – in Yoga 'static' does not mean 'inactive' or passive.

Almost every posture presented will describe a dynamic as well as a static version. If you are a beginner, start with the dynamic version before attempting the static version. This allows the body to become accustomed to the motion of moving into and recovering out of a posture, and also helps to prepare the body and mind for the posture by warming up the area/s of the body that is/are involved.

As you become more advanced in your practice, you will be able to hold postures for longer periods of time.

The basic criterion for holding a posture is that you feel comfortable in it. It is important to discern the difference between constructive stretching and the pain of pushing your body too far.

Always enter into and recover out of postures slowly and with care (perhaps doing the dynamic version first, even if it is just twice or three times, as preparation).

Make sure you are able to breathe easily while in a posture. It is best to repeat a static posture twice or three times, holding the posture for a shorter period, rather than straining to hold the position in one long stretch.

Postures and counter-postures

Each posture needs to be balanced by another posture that either bends the body in the opposite direction or returns the body to a position of symmetry. This allows the body to restore a state of equilibrium and to gain the full benefit from the postures. If you experience discomfort after doing a posture, remedy the problem by moving into the counter-posture, whether it be a dynamic, a static or a resting posture.

The counter-posture is an easier posture than the original posture and can take the form of a rest pose, especially for beginners. Certain postures presented include suggestions for counter-postures on the same page.

Hold the counter-posture for a third of the time that you held the initial posture, or execute the counter-posture dynamically. Postures that particularly require counter-postures include back bends, twists, side bends and inverted postures.

- Back bends are to be followed by a forward bend.
- Twists and side bends are to be followed by a symmetrical posture in a forward bend (the rest pose in Apanasana is also appropriate). Also, after carrying out a twist or a side bend on one side of the body, return to a symmetrical position before twisting or bending the other way. This returns the spine to a comfortably aligned position, as a starting point for bending in the other direction. (Take care not to do a back bend directly before or after a twist or side bend, as it can be dangerous for the spine.)
- Inverted postures are to be followed by a rest pose, such as the Child's pose or Savasana (the Corpse pose). This allows the blood flow to return to normal in the body. Do not stand up too quickly after holding an inverted posture, such as the headstand, as this may cause dizziness. Remain in the rest pose for at least a third of the time you held the inverted pose, or until you feel ready to recover.

THE POSTURE SUMMARY CHART

On pages 38–39 you will find a summary chart of all the postures in this book (excluding the warming-up and meditation postures) to help you devise a Yoga session. The postures are divided into five main posture groups: neutral, forward bend, back bend, side bend; and twist. These five groups are further divided into: sitting, standing, standing balance, hand balance, inverted, resting, and counter-posture or rest options.

In order to facilitate easy reference, only one version of each posture is depicted – simplified versions are presented in Chapter 5, The Postures.

Once you have selected your postures, turn to the relevant pages to read the detailed instructions, and follow the gradual progression from beginner to advanced.

You'll find that most of the postures have preparatory exercises that should be mastered comfortably before moving on to a more advanced version.

The postures on the chart are graded for difficulty level: ☀ is suitable for beginners, while ☀ ☀ ☀ ☀ indicates the most advanced level.

The order of a session

A general guideline is:
1. warm-up
2. simple postures
3. more challenging postures and inverted postures
4. rest posture/counter-posture
5. balance posture
6. rest pose
7. breathing practice
8. meditation.

Warm up sufficiently

Include two to five warm-up exercises, both general and specific to the respective postures. You'll find details of warm-up exercises on pages 40–57.

This will ensure that the relevant area/s of your body are well prepared for the safe execution of the desired posture.

Simple and more challenging postures

These may include postures from different groups or may focus on a particular posture group.

Select between two to six postures; start with forward bends, as they require flexibility. Move onto back bends, which require strength, when your body is well warmed up.

Remember that it is not necessary to include postures from each category – you can choose to focus on a particular category on one day and another on another day.

You can also repeat postures – if you use a forward bend near the beginning of a session, you can use the same forward bend later as a counter-posture to a back bend.

Rest postures

Include rest postures at least three or four times during the session to allow your body to rest between postures. You can also begin a session with a rest pose in order to prepare the mind and body for a relaxed approach to the postures.

Counter-postures

It is important that you alternate posture and counter-posture throughout the session – hold the counter-posture for a third of the time that you held the final static posture.

You can do two or three postures in the same group before doing a counter-posture. For example, if you are working on back bends, warm up with simple dynamic and static versions, such as Bhujangasana (the Cobra) and Salabhasana (the Locust), followed by a more challenging posture such as Dhanurasana (the Bow). Then move into a forward bend.

To allow your session to flow from one posture into the next, try to group sitting postures and standing postures, so that you are not constantly moving from a sitting to a standing position. You may start off sitting, then do a few standing postures, then return to sitting, or the other way around, to make your session flow as much as possible in order to avoid discomfort.

Balance postures

Choose a balance in a position for which your body has warmed up. For example, if you have included Baddha Konasana, you will find Vrksasana easier to achieve.

If you focus on forward bends, you could balance in Navasana or a more advanced balance such as Virabhadrasana.

Concluding rest pose

Your session should end with a rest pose, such as Savasana (the Corpse), for 5–10 minutes.

You'll find details of breathing and meditation on pages 150–155. These can also be done at any time of the day, even when you're not practising your other Yoga postures.

Once you have selected a sequence of postures that works for you, repeat this session over a few weeks or months to gauge your progress. This way you will reap maximum benefits from your practice, rather than doing a new posture every day.

The timing of your Yoga session

Set aside a minimum of 15–30 minutes for a session, although an hour and a half is the recommended time to be able to include a variation of postures as well as relaxation, breathing practices and meditation. If you only have little time, such as 20–30 minutes, choose fewer postures and focus on them, rather than rushing through too many.

Ideas for sessions of different lengths

15-minute session
- 10 minutes – Surya Namaskar (Sun Salutation) and rest pose in Vajrasana (the Child's pose) or Savasana
- 5 minutes – breathing and meditation

30-minute session
- 5 minutes – warm-up
- 20 minutes – forward bend (dynamic/static), back bend (dynamic/static), forward bend (static), twist, forward bend, one/two standing poses (dynamic/static), rest pose
- 5 minutes – breathing and meditation

1-hour session or longer
- 5–10 minutes – warm-up
- 35 minutes – forward bend (dynamic\static), back bend (dynamic\static), forward bend (static), twist, forward bend, one or two standing poses (dynamic\static), balance, rest pose, inverted pose, rest pose
- 15 minutes – breathing and meditation
- Longer periods of meditation will be of benefit (such as 30–45 minute meditation practice) and can be added to a Yoga session or done at any time of the day, such as in the early morning or in the evening.

A sample 30-minute Yoga session

- Warm up for five minutes
- Twenty minutes of postures:

Forward bend		☼ – ☼☼☼ Pascimottanasana p72
Back bend		☼ – ☼☼ Bidalasana p82
Forward bend		☼☼ – ☼☼☼☼ Supta Baddha Konasana p69
Twist		☼ – ☼☼☼ Jathara Parivartanasana p100
Forward bend		☼ – ☼☼☼ Upavista Konasana p74
Standing postures	☼ Tadasana p108	☼☼ Vrkshasana p126
Rest		Savasana p148

Five minutes of breathing and meditation

THE POSTURE SUMMARY CHART

Posture groups	Neutral		Forward bend		
Sitting or lying	☀ – ☀☀☀ Vajrasana p64	☀ Dandasana p73	☀☀ – ☀☀☀ Supta Vajrasana p64	☀☀ – ☀☀☀ Pascimottanasana p72	
			☀ – ☀☀☀ Supta Baddha Konasana p69	☀ – ☀☀☀ Janu Sirshasana p70	
	☀ – ☀☀☀ Baddha Konasana p68		☀ – ☀☀☀ Upavista Konasana p74	☀☀ – ☀☀☀☀ Paripurna Navasana p78	
	☀ – ☀☀ Gomukhasana p66		☀ – ☀☀☀☀ Akarna Dhanurasana p76		
Standing	☀ Tadasana p108	☀☀ Virabhadrasana 2 p116	☀ Utkatasana p109	☀ – ☀☀☀ Uttanasana p110	☀☀ – ☀☀☀ Parsva Uttanasana p112
Standing balance	☀☀ Vrksasana p126	☀☀ – ☀☀☀☀ Utthita Hasta Padangusthasana p131	☀☀☀ Garudasana p127	☀☀☀ Virabhadrasana 3 p128	
Hand balance	☀☀ Chaturangsana p132	☀☀ – ☀☀☀☀ Mayurasana p134	☀☀ – ☀☀☀☀ Adho Mukha Vrkshasana p135	☀☀ – ☀☀☀☀ Bakasana p134	
Inverted	☀☀ – ☀☀☀ Salamba Sirshasana p142		☀☀ – ☀☀☀ Sarvangasana p138	☀☀ – ☀☀☀☀ Halasana p140	
Rest poses	Savasana p148		Supta Vajrasana p149	Apanasana p149	
Counter-posture or rest options	Samasthiti p108		Hanging forward bend p107	Viparita Karani against a wall p139	Halasana over a chair p141

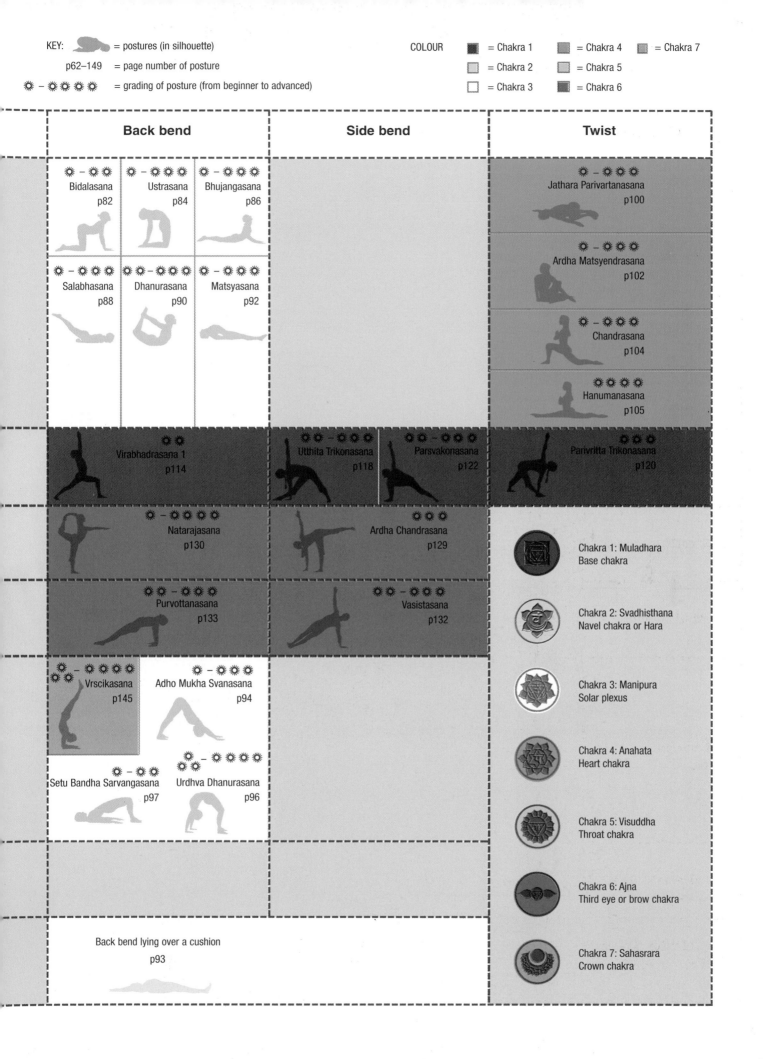

KEY: = postures (in silhouette)

p62–149 = page number of posture

☀ – ☀☀☀☀ = grading of posture (from beginner to advanced)

COLOUR ◼ = Chakra 1 ◼ = Chakra 4 ◼ = Chakra 7
◻ = Chakra 2 ◻ = Chakra 5
◻ = Chakra 3 ◼ = Chakra 6

Back bend			Side bend		Twist
☀ – ☀☀ Bidalasana p82	☀ – ☀☀☀ Ustrasana p84	☀ – ☀☀☀ Bhujangasana p86			☀ – ☀☀☀ Jathara Parivartanasana p100
☀ – ☀☀☀ Salabhasana p88	☀☀ – ☀☀☀ Dhanurasana p90	☀ – ☀☀☀ Matsyasana p92			☀ – ☀☀☀ Ardha Matsyendrasana p102
					☀ – ☀☀☀ Chandrasana p104
					☀☀☀☀ Hanumanasana p105
☀☀ Virabhadrasana 1 p114			☀☀ – ☀☀☀ Utthita Trikonasana p118	☀☀ – ☀☀☀ Parsvakonasana p122	☀☀☀ Parivritta Trikonasana p120
☀ – ☀☀☀☀ Natarajasana p130			☀☀☀ Ardha Chandrasana p129		
☀☀ – ☀☀☀ Purvottanasana p133			☀☀ – ☀☀☀ Vasistasana p132		
☀☀ – ☀☀☀☀ Vrscikasana p145	☀ – ☀☀☀ Adho Mukha Svanasana p94				
☀ – ☀☀ Setu Bandha Sarvangasana p97	☀☀ – ☀☀☀☀ Urdhva Dhanurasana p96				
Back bend lying over a cushion p93					

Chakra 1: Muladhara
Base chakra

Chakra 2: Svadhisthana
Navel chakra or Hara

Chakra 3: Manipura
Solar plexus

Chakra 4: Anahata
Heart chakra

Chakra 5: Visuddha
Throat chakra

Chakra 6: Ajna
Third eye or brow chakra

Chakra 7: Sahasrara
Crown chakra

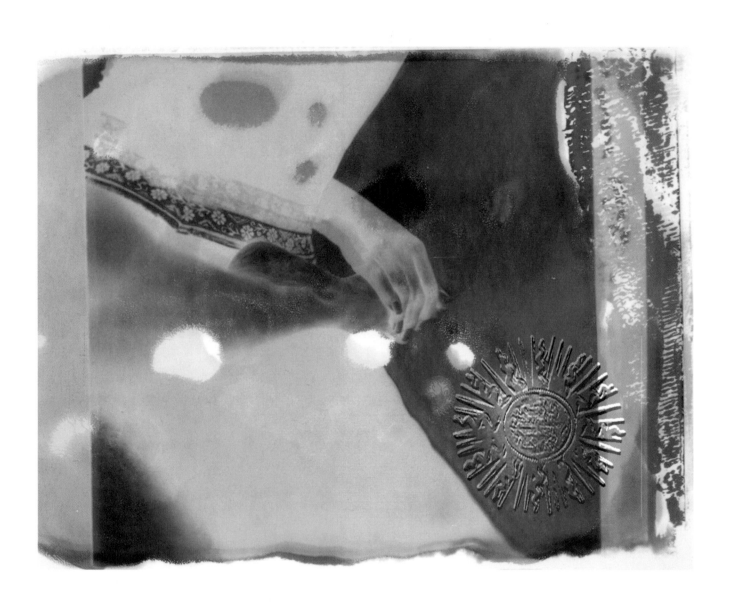

CHAPTER 4

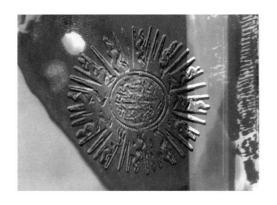

WARMING UP

Warming up

One of the reasons it is important to warm up the body is because this focuses attention on the breath and encourages deeper breathing to increase the oxygen intake, which in turn enhances energy levels and concentration in preparation for Yoga. These exercises also serve to wake up the body in the morning or wind it down at the end of a busy day.

Blood circulation to the extremities of the body is improved by warming up, which is helpful for sensing body alignment and full extension in postures. Warming up also helps prepare the body for the attainment of postures with greater ease and prevents injury; in addition it reduces stiffness after practising Yoga, as increased oxygen supply and circulation to the muscles reduces the accumulation of lactic acid in the muscles.

A better posture and increased awareness of your body alignment are further benefits of warming up, and the session assists the mind to focus on the Yoga to be practised.

You'll find that warm-up exercises are often useful for quick and effective relief at any time of day and in any location.

For example, simple stretches can be done in an office or while travelling on an aeroplane, in order to relax and reduce muscular tension, relieve fatigue, stimulate blood circulation and generally increase energy levels.

A warm-up routine involves either the Sun Salutation or a series of preliminary exercises for each part of the body, from head to toe. You will probably not have time in a single session to do all the exercises. The idea is, over time, to try out the exercises and choose the ones that you like or feel that you need the most.

Cautions in devising a warm-up

If you have a past (or current) injury, a problem or stiffness in a particular area of your body, it is advisable to incorporate warm-up exercises for the respective area/s. Your Yoga teacher may notice stiffness or tightness in your body that you're not aware of, and recommend that you see a health practitioner for assessment.

If you are injured or have a medical condition, consult your health practitioner and Yoga teacher before practising any of the warm-up exercises – they may advise you to focus on certain ones and to avoid others. If you have chosen to focus on a particular posture group or a single posture, make sure that you also focus the warm-up on the area or areas of your body which are relevant to the respective group of postures.

Devising a warm-up routine

Some people like to create a ritual of the warm-up session, which will allow it to become familiar to the body.

This familiarity in the warm-up routine allows the Yoga practitioner to concentrate on more mindful use of the body; a ritual beginning sets the tone for more focused attention thereafter.

To devise a personalized warm-up ritual (from head to toe, or focusing on a specific area of the body), try out each exercise over a period of time. Then select the ones with which you feel comfortable and feel you most need. You can order the exercises as you choose.

You may need to add into your ritual specific preparatory exercises for specific postures that you have chosen to practise in your session.

Head to toe warm-up

All movements are to be executed in a slow, gentle and controlled manner, co-ordinating breath with movement (unless otherwise specified). Breathing is to be slow and controlled.

Caution: Never force any movement or stretch as you may injure yourself.

Starting positions

The warm-up exercises that follow can be done either sitting or standing.

Starting position for sitting

Sit upright, on the ground or on a cushion on the ground, with your spine extended. Cross your legs in a comfortable position. Rest your hands on your thighs or knees.

Starting position for standing

Stand upright with your spine extended, arms at your sides, legs parallel and straight or slightly bent. The feet are together or hip distance apart.

Head and face warm-ups

The following exercises help to relax the face before Yoga, which is often an area in which we hold tension, in many cases without even being aware of it.

Eyes

1–4. Keeping your head centred and still, focus your eyes up, down, side to side and diagonally up and down.

Circle your eyes two or three times clockwise, then repeat the action anti-clockwise.

Close your eyes. Rub your hands together and then cup your warmed palms over your eyes. Open your eyes into the darkness and absorb the darkness into your eye sockets for two or three breaths. Close your eyes as you release your hands and then open your eyes, allowing them to come to rest gently on whatever happens to be lying in front of them.

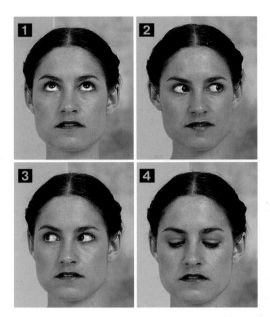

Facial muscles

1. Tighten all your facial muscles, closing your eyes tightly and pursing your lips.
2. Now do the opposite. Open your eyes and mouth as wide as possible and stick out your tongue.

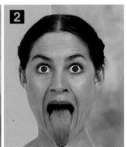

Neck warm-ups

These exercises will relax your neck before Yoga. Do not do them if you have a neck injury or if you feel uncomfortable.

Turning the head

A. Inhaling, turn your head to the right side as far as you can. Exhaling, return your head to the front. Repeat to the left. Alternate the movement two or three times in a flowing manner, keeping your chin parallel to the ground.

Back of the neck

B. Exhale, then lower your chin down to your chest. Hold for a minimum of two breaths. To recover, inhale, returning your head to the upright position.

Front of the neck

C. Inhale and raise your chin, stretching the front of your neck. Hold for one or two breaths. Exhaling, lower your chin to your chest and hold for one or two breaths.

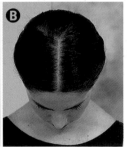

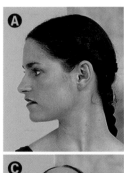

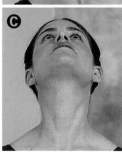

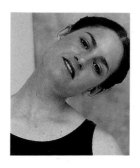

Side neck stretches

Exhale and lower your ear towards your shoulder.

Press down in the opposite shoulder to increase the stretch up the side of your neck. Keep your head and eyes facing forward. Hold for one or two breaths.

To recover, exhale slowly, allowing your chin to lower to your chest as your head hangs forwards into a centred position. While inhaling, return your head to the upright position. Repeat on the other side.

Full head rolls

Slowly roll your head in a circular pathway. Exhale and lower your chin to your chest.

While inhaling, roll your head to the right side and to the centre position, facing up with your chin raised.

While exhaling, roll your head to the left side and to the centre position with your head lowered and your chin to your chest. Take care to keep the back of your neck extended throughout and make sure you move smoothly, in a flowing manner.

Repeat once or twice in a clockwise direction, and then perform the full head rolls in an anti-clockwise direction.

Shoulder and arm warm-ups

In each of the warm-up exercises below, remember to repeat the circling motions of your arms in both directions.

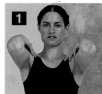
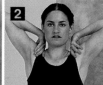
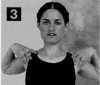
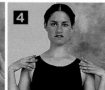

Shoulder circles

1–2. Inhaling, move your shoulders forwards and up towards your ears.
3–4. Exhaling, move your shoulders backwards and press them down.
Repeat two or three times.

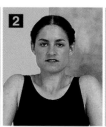
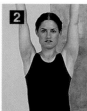
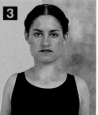
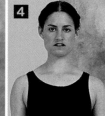

Upper arm circles

1–2. Place your hands on your shoulders, with bent elbows. Circle your elbows, keeping your shoulders pressed down. Inhaling, move them forward and up.
3–4. Exhaling, move them backwards and down. Repeat two to four times.

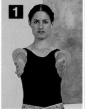
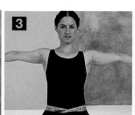
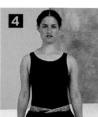

Full arm circles

1. Move your arms in a circular pathway, keeping your arms fully extended.
2. Inhaling, move the arms forward and up.
3–4. Exhaling, move the arms backwards and down. Repeat two to four times.

Wrist warm-ups

1–2. Extend your arms out in front of you. Circle your wrists and hands two to three times in each direction.

Hand warm-ups

Extend your arms in front of you. Start shaking your hands, working gradually up your arm for a good 'shaking out'.

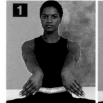
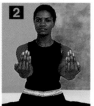

Foot and ankle warm-ups

Sit upright, with legs extended, arms at your sides and hands on the ground next to your hips. Check that your weight is evenly distributed over the two sides of your buttocks.

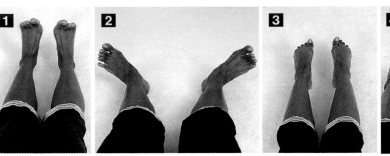

1–4. Start with both your feet flexed. Rotate your feet and ankles outward three times, then rotate them inward three times. If you wish to do this warm-up standing, use one foot at a time.

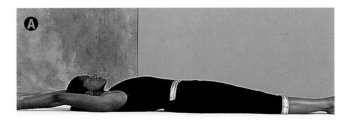

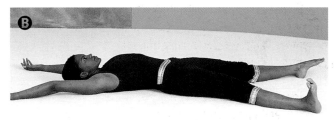

Body warm-ups

For these exercises, lie flat on your back with your arms stretched up next to your ears and legs stretched out in front of you.

Body stretching

A. Inhaling, extend your legs and arms, so that your entire body is stretched – legs and arms reach in opposite directions. Exhaling, relax. Repeat, stretching only the right side of your body, then only the left side. Restore symmetry by stretching both sides together again.

Stretch and curl

1. Inhaling, stretch out your entire body.
2. Exhaling, curl your body into a tight ball, bringing your knees to your forehead and hugging your legs with your arms. Repeat two or three times. This exercise warms your spine and strengthens your abdominal muscles.

Diagonal body stretching

B. Open your arms and legs into 'V' shapes. Inhaling, extend your right arm and left leg. Exhale and relax. Repeat, stretching your left arm and right leg. Then repeat stretching both arms and both legs together to restore symmetry.

Rolling ball

Bend your knees and hug them into your chest, with hands holding underneath your bent knees. Round your spine and tuck your chin into your chest throughout.

1–2. Initiate a backwards and forwards rocking motion, reaching your legs overhead and swinging forwards again. This motion helps to alleviate stiffness and align the vertebrae. **Caution: Do not do if you are not able to round your spine. If you feel any discomfort, stop.**

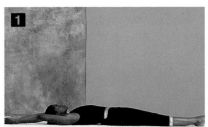

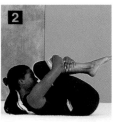

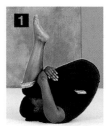

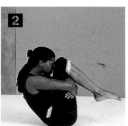

Leg and hip warm-ups

A. The starting position is on your back with your legs held together, outstretched and parallel, knees locked and feet flexed. Arms rest on the ground, alongside your body with palms facing down, unless otherwise specified.

Avoid arching your lower back or raising your buttocks during the exercises. This is achieved by feeling as if you are pressing your abdominal muscles to the ground.

Keep your head on the ground, unless otherwise specified.

All movement is co-ordinated with the breath, taking care not to rush or jerk any movements.

You may find a strap useful to assist in holding leg raises while working to increase your flexibility. If you do use a strap, sling it around the sole of your foot or around your ankle and hold onto it with both hands.

Caution: If you are pregnant, keep your legs apart in all exercises, so that you don't apply pressure on your abdomen. Stay with the simpler exercises, particularly after the first three months of pregnancy.

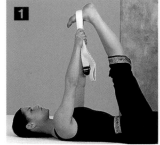
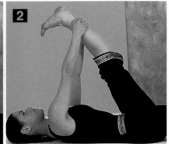

Single leg raises (extended version)

1. Raise your right leg.
2. Take hold of your ankle or toes with both hands or with a strap slung around your foot. Keep both legs extended, with your feet flexed. Hold for two to six breaths. Repeat with your left leg.

Double leg raises

C. Inhaling, raise both legs, keeping them pressed together and extended. Exhaling, lower both legs back to the starting position. Repeat two to 10 times.

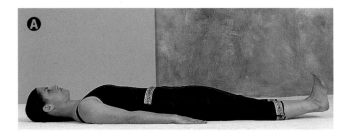

Single leg raises

B. Inhaling, raise your right leg as high as you can.
Exhaling, lower the leg back to the starting position.
Repeat the raise using your left leg. Alternate the legs two to four times.

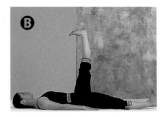

Caution: If you experience discomfort in the lower back, or have weak abdominal muscles, keep one knee bent with the sole of the foot on the ground while the other leg is raised.

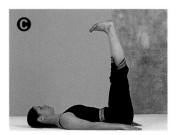

Caution: Only attempt to do double leg raises when you have developed enough strength in your abdominal and lower back muscles to support the exercise. If you are struggling to prevent your lower back from arching or your buttocks from lifting off the ground, stay with single leg raises until your strength increases.

Double leg raises (extended version)

Raise both legs as above, holding as for the single leg raises. Gently pull your legs towards you, keeping them extended and your spine and buttocks in contact with the ground. Hold for three to six breaths.

Inner thigh and hip flex

1. Start with both legs raised. Bend your knees, turning your legs out so that the soles of your feet touch and your knees open out to the sides. Hold your feet or ankles in your hands, easing your feet in towards you. Hold for two to six breaths.
2. Open your legs out to the sides, while pressing your hands on your inner thighs. Hold for two to six breaths.

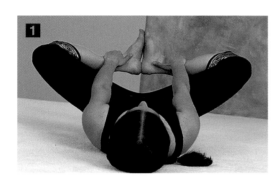

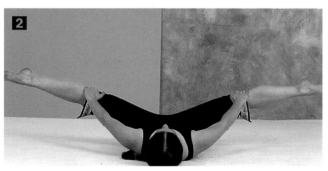

Thigh stretch

D. Lie on your abdomen, with your forehead resting on your right hand. The legs are straight and held together. Bend your left leg and hold your foot with your left hand. Ease

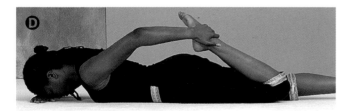

your heel in towards your buttocks until you feel a stretch in the left thigh muscle. Try to keep your knees touching throughout. Hold for three to six breaths, then repeat with your right leg.

The wind-relieving postures

The following postures function as rest postures after any of the leg and hip warm-ups. Make sure you don't raise your buttocks from the ground.

The asymmetrical version

E. Bend your right leg and hug your knee over your abdomen, with your foot relaxed. Your left leg is extended on the ground and held parallel with your foot flexed. Hold for three to six breaths, then repeat with your left leg. Always use your right leg first, as this gives a gentle squeeze to the beginning of the large intestine, helping digestion in the antigravity direction of this portion of the intestine.

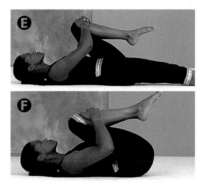

The symmetrical version

F. Complete this posture as you would the asymmetrical version, except bring both legs, one by one, to the chest.

The open-legged version

G. This version of the wind-relieving posture works on the mobility of the hips, while the two earlier versions worked on the abdominal and lower back area. Practise the open-legged version if you are pregnant.

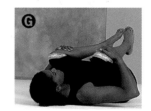

Standing warm-ups

The starting position, unless otherwise specified, is upright, with your legs and feet together and your arms at your sides.

Spinal curling

1. Exhaling, start relaxing forwards by lowering your head. Then, vertebra for vertebra, relax your spine, relaxing your neck, shoulders, arms, chest.
2. Finally, relax your lower back so that your entire spine is rounded and hanging forwards. Bend your knees so that there is no strain placed on your spine.

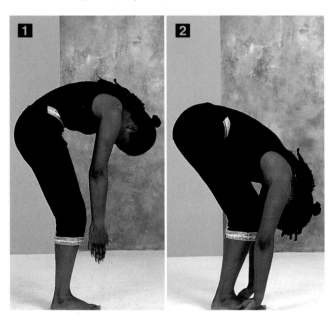

Inhaling, slowly uncurl, reversing the path taken on the exhalation. Keep your abdomen pressed lightly against your spine, breathing into your chest. Repeat two to four times.

Side bends

1. Stand with your hands on your waist (if you're sitting, place your hand on the ground for support).
2. Inhaling, raise your right arm, placing it next to your right ear.
3. Exhaling, bend over to the left side, stretching your right side. Keep your right arm extended and next to your ear throughout. Hold for two or three breaths.

Recover on an inhalation, reversing the path as you return to an upright, centred position. Repeat to the other side. To restore symmetry in your body, relax forward as for spinal curling and hold for two or three breaths.

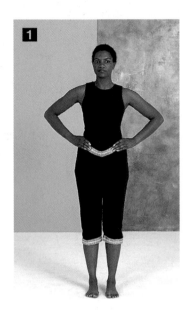

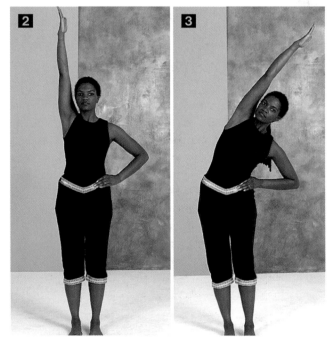

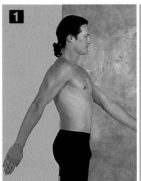
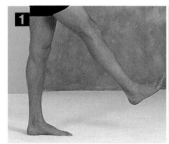

Arm swings

1–2. With your abdomen lightly pressed against your spine throughout, swing your arms forwards and backwards (in a walking motion) keeping your arms even in height to the front and back.

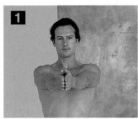
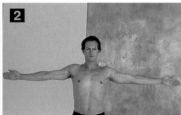

Arm opening

1–2. Open and close both your arms, keeping them at shoulder height.

Torso twists

A. Gently twist your torso from side to side, taking your head with you. Bend your knees slightly to allow for the gentle twisting motion.

Caution: Don't be too rigorous with your swings. If you have a back problem, take care with spinal twists or avoid them. Always twist very gently and with care.

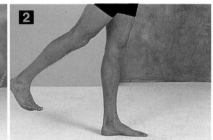

Leg swings

1–2. Place your hands on your hips. Shift your weight over onto your left leg and swing your right leg like a pendulum (forwards and backwards), gradually swinging your leg higher with each swing, while keeping the height of your raised leg even to the front and the back. Keep both legs straight throughout.

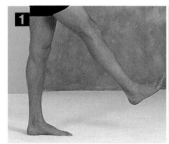

Arm and leg swings

1–2. Add arm swings to the leg swings by swinging your arms forwards and backwards in a walking motion. The outstretched leg moves in opposition to the arm of the same side. Do not raise your arms above shoulder height. Then shake out your legs and arms.

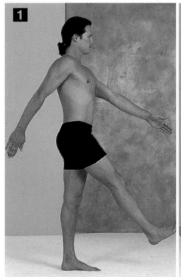
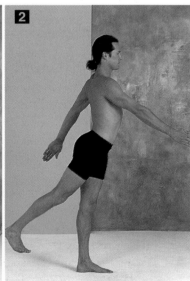
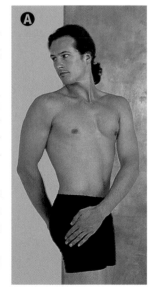

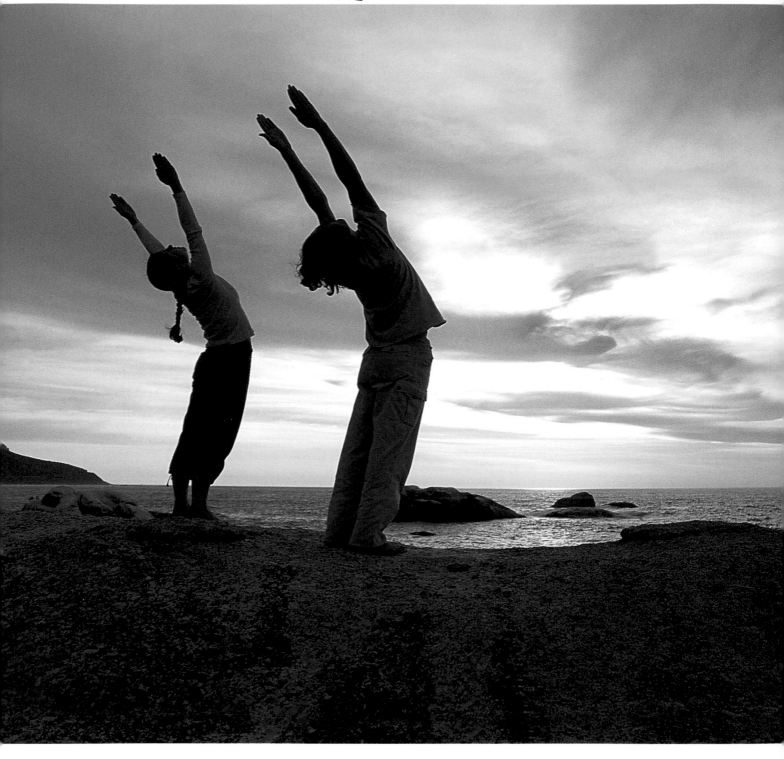

'Surya' means sun and 'Namaskar' refers to a greeting or salutation. The sun salutation is a moving sequence made up of a combination of Yoga postures. It originated as a series of prostrations carried out to the rising sun. Saluting the sun is a gesture of gratefulness for the sun's lighting, brightening, warming and energizing nature and effect on our lives.

Surya

Namaskar offers an effective way to limber up, stretch, tone and strengthen the entire body and spine. Each posture in the sequence is arranged in such a way that postures stretching and opening the chest area are followed by ones that close or contract the chest. This frees the respiratory system and encourages deeper breathing. Surya Namaskar increases the blood circulation to the whole body. This increased blood circulation, together with the increased oxygen supply as a result of deeper breathing, revitalizes and energizes the body and focuses the mind.

The sequence is to be carried out in a smooth, flowing manner from one posture to the next. Benefits are gained not only from the postures themselves, but also from the transitional movement between postures. The co-ordination of breath with movement is particularly helpful in this regard and when practised with flow, a sense of poise and gracefulness will be achieved.

It is an excellent warm-up, as it offers an effective way to wake up and energize the body at the start of a session. It can also be included at any stage in the Yoga session, or used on its own if you only have a short time to practice.

The Sun Salutation is suitable for all age-groups and levels of fitness, if you take care to stay with the version with which you are comfortable. The three versions presented here progress in degree of difficulty. If you have any spinal problem, take care to keep your legs bent on forward bends and to take care on back bends.

Caution: This sequence is not recommended for people with high blood pressure or a heart condition or in the case of any eye or ear condition where inversion is not advisable. It is also not advised for pregnant women.

To gain maximum benefits, practise the Sun Salutation regularly as part of your session. Start with two or three rounds and work up to 12 rounds. One round (in the beginner and intermediate versions) is made up of the entire sequence carried out twice, first using the right leg in steps 4 and 9, then using the left leg.

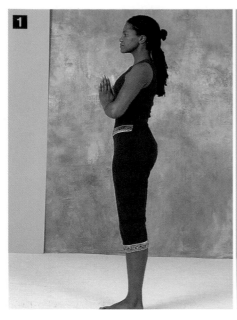 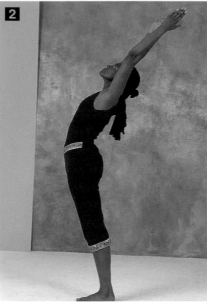 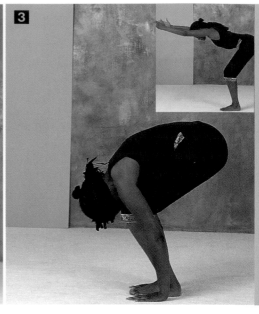

Beginner's version ☼

1. Stand upright, with spine extended, legs straight and feet together. The arms are in the Prayer pose, with elbows pointing to the sides and palms together, positioned against your breastbone. Your weight is evenly distributed over both legs and feet.

2. Inhaling, raise and extend your arms overhead and bend slightly backwards in your upper back as you reach up and backwards with your arms. Part your hands so the palms face each other and your arms are parallel and next to your ears. Your head faces upwards, following the line of movement; keep the back of your neck extended.

3. Exhaling, reach your arms and fingers up, forwards and down, keeping arms extended and next to your ears. Head and neck remain in line with the spine to keep your back straight as you bend forwards from your hips (see insert). When you can bend no further without rounding your spine, place your hands flat on the ground next to your feet, bending your knees as necessary. Tuck in your head so that your forehead aims towards your knees or shins.

4. Inhaling, extend your right leg behind you, placing the top of your right foot and your right knee on the ground, with toes pointing behind you. The left leg bends so that the heel is positioned under the knee, creating a right angle. Sink into your right hip as you feel the stretch across the front of your right hip. Look up, stretching the front of your neck and raising your chin.

5. Retaining your breath, bring your left leg to join your right leg, so that your weight is on all fours, with the knees slightly behind your hips. Neck and head are in line with the rest of your spine, so that eyes look down to the ground between your hands. Arms remain straight. Take care to keep 'lifted out of' your shoulders to avoid straining in your shoulders and neck.

6. Exhaling, lower your chest and forehead to the ground (this is the Caterpillar pose). Keep the elbows in at your sides as your arms bend.

7. Inhaling, straighten your legs and slide your chest along the ground until your hips touch the ground. Stretch forwards and up through your head, raising your body off the ground

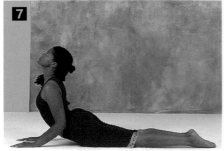 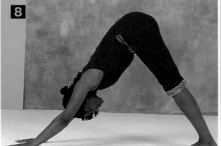 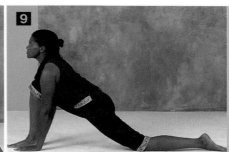

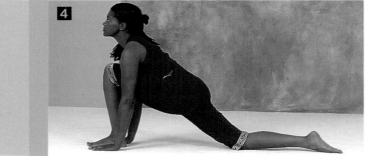

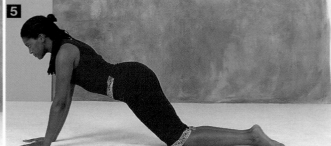

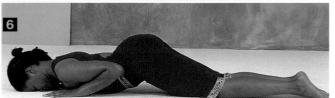

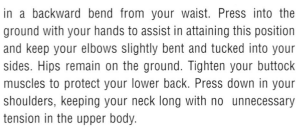

in a backward bend from your waist. Press into the ground with your hands to assist in attaining this position and keep your elbows slightly bent and tucked into your sides. Hips remain on the ground. Tighten your buttock muscles to protect your lower back. Press down in your shoulders, keeping your neck long with no unnecessary tension in the upper body.

8. Exhaling, slightly lower your chest while curling your toes under. Push up and back with your arms while raising your hips until your body forms an inverted 'V'. Body weight is evenly distributed between hands and feet – try to get your heels on the ground. The knees are straight or slightly bent, the head is between the arms (arms are next to the ears). Arch your back (particularly the lower back) by reaching up through the tailbone as high as you can.

9. Inhaling, bend your right leg, bringing it forwards and placing it between your hands, while lowering the left knee to the ground. Release your toes, returning to step 4, with the right leg forward this time. The right leg forms a right angle, with your heel under your knee.

10. Exhaling, bring your left leg up so that it is next to your right foot, returning to step 3.

11. Inhaling, reach your arms forward and place them next to your ears (see insert). Return to the upright position by reversing the path taken in step 2. Keep your arms next to your ears so your neck and head remain in line with the spine; the back is straight. Straighten your knees once you are upright and bend slightly back, as for step 2.

12. Exhaling, return your hands to the Prayer pose.

Note: Your hands remain in the same position on the floor from steps 3 to 10. Repeat using your left leg in steps 4 and 9, and your right leg for steps 5 and 10.

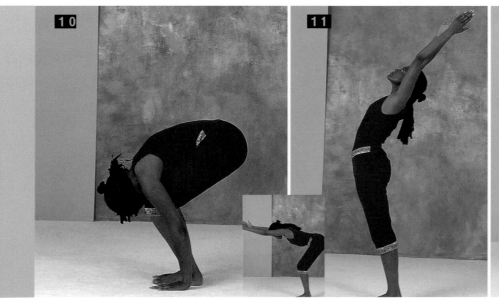

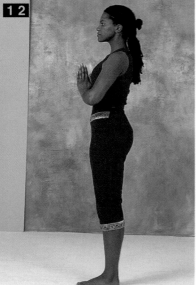

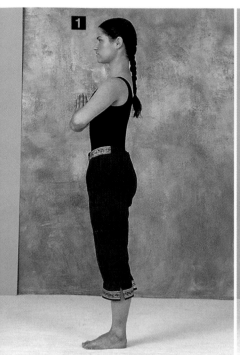

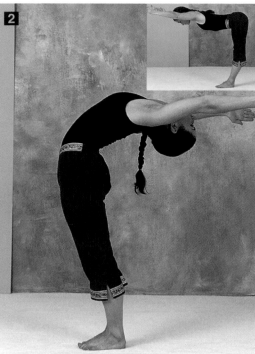

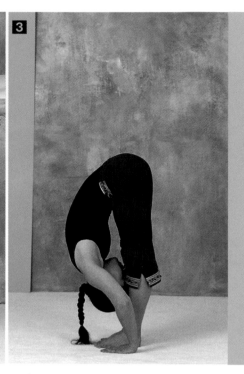

Intermediate / Advanced version ☀ ☀

Follow the instructions as for the Beginner's version, making changes as follows:

1. Stand upright with your hands in the Prayer pose (elbows pointing out and the palms together).

2. Inhaling, move into a back bend, allowing your head to look up and back, following the line of movement.

3. Exhaling, move into a forward bend, keeping your legs straight with your knees locked (if you need to, you can bend your knees slightly).

4. Inhaling, extend your right leg behind you, curling the toes of your right foot under and keeping the right leg straight with the knee locked.

5. Retaining your breath, bring your left leg back to join the right, balancing on your hands and toes (the Plank pose). Legs are together and hips in line with the body; neck and head are in line with the spine; eyes look to the ground between or just beyond your hands. Arms remain straight. Keep lifted out of your shoulders, to avoid straining in your shoulders and neck.

6. Exhaling, lower your knees, chest and forehead to the ground (the Caterpillar pose). Keep your elbows in at your sides as your arms bend.

7. Inhaling, bend as far into the back bend as you can, keeping your arms slightly bent and your hips on the ground. Because this posture compresses the lumbar region, you need to exercise caution. Ask your Yoga teacher for advice.

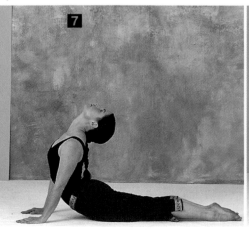

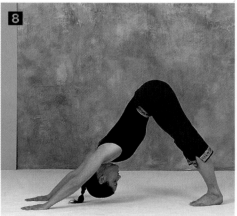

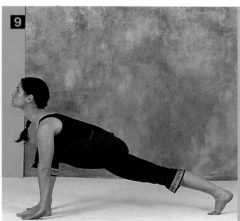

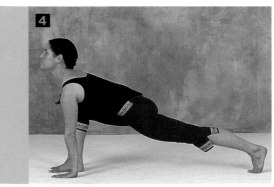 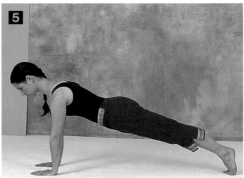 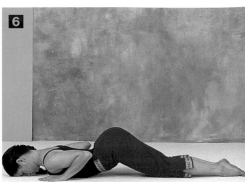

8. Exhaling, push yourself back into the V-shaped dog stretch as in the beginner's version (step 8).

9. Inhaling, bend your right leg, bringing it forward and placing it between your hands, as you return to step 4, with the opposite leg now brought forward. Keep your left leg extended with toes curled under.

10. Exhaling, bring your left foot to be placed next to your right foot. Both legs are straightened in the forward bend, with knees locked and hands flat on the ground alongside your feet, as for step 3.

11. Inhaling, reach your arms forward, placing them next to your ears, then recover to the upright position in the back bend as for step 2. Take care to keep your arms next to your ears so that the neck and head are in line with the rest of the spine and the back is straight.

12. Exhaling, return to the Prayer pose, step 1.

Note: Try not to adjust the position of the hands on the floor from step 3 through to 10.

Repeat using your left leg in steps 4 and 9, and the right leg for steps 5 and 10.

To increase the intensity of the Sun Salutation for a more strenuous work-out, hold each of the 12 positions for two to six breaths, before moving on to the next. For step 5, breathe while holding the Plank.

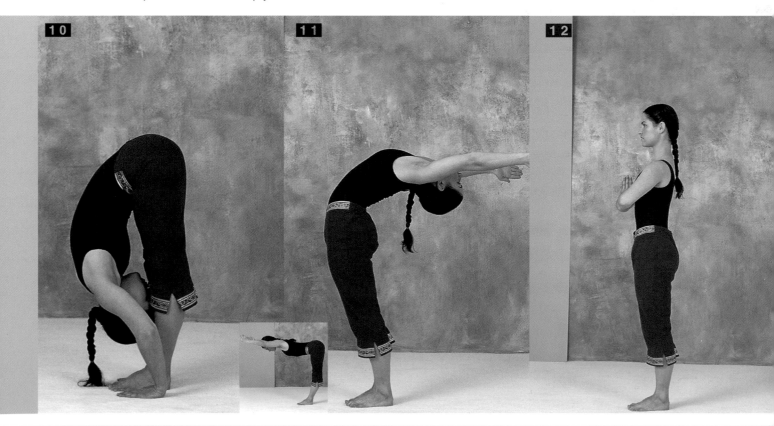

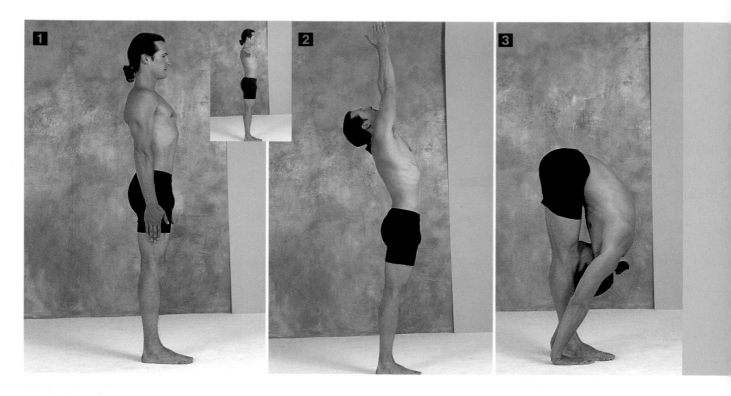

Advanced version ☀ ☀ ☀

This is another strenuous option, with 11 instead of 12 positions in the sequence.

1. The starting position is upright, with spine extended, arms at your sides, chest open, legs straight and feet together.
2. Inhaling, extend and raise your arms up sideways (see insert) to bring your palms to touch overhead. Eyes look up to your hands.
3. Exhaling, reach your arms forwards, keeping your arms next to your ears and spine straight as you bend forwards from your hips until you can bend no further without rounding your spine. Then place your hands on the ground alongside you

feet. Legs remain straight (if you need to, bend them slightly). Eyes look toward your navel.

4. Inhaling, reach forward with your head, extending your spine as you do so, so that your eyes look out to the ground in front of you.
5. Exhaling, spring back with your feet (see insert), landing on

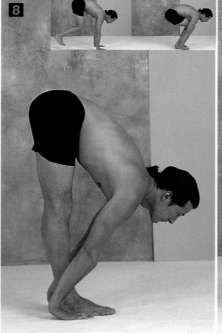

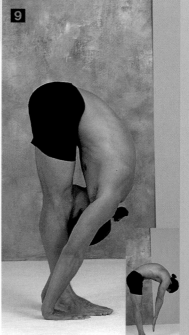

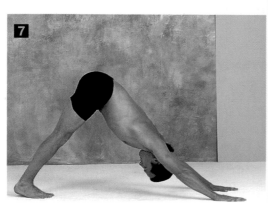

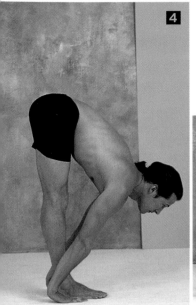

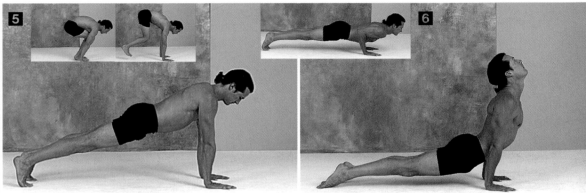

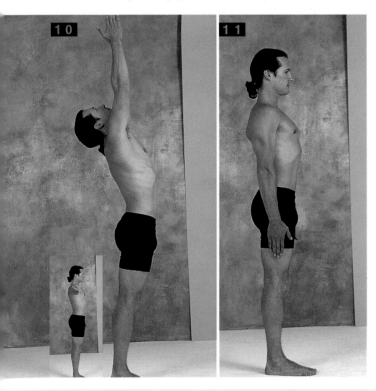

your toes, with your body in the Plank pose (hips in line with the lower and upper body, with legs straight and knees locked). Keep your head reaching forward, so your neck is in line with the rest of your spine.

6. Inhaling, bend your elbows, lowering your chest between your arms (see insert) in preparation for the inhalation. Inhale, straightening your elbows as you reach forwards and up with your head, chest and chin; you are now in a back bend, with eyes looking straight up. Release your toes to point behind you and shift your weight forwards. Keep your hips raised off the ground.

7. Exhaling, bend your elbows as you slightly lower your chest in preparation for the exhalation. Exhale, straighten your elbows, raise your hips and push your weight back – you are now in an inverted 'V' shape, with your weight evenly distributed between your hands and feet. Try to get your heels on the ground. Arch your lower and upper back. Eyes look toward your navel. Hold this position for about five breaths.

8. Inhaling, spring your feet to land back between your hands, bending your knees to soften your landing (see inserts). As you spring, reach forwards with your head, so that your spine remains slightly extended and your eyes look out to the ground in front of you. Straighten, returning to step 4.

9. Exhaling, return to step 3, in a full forward bend, with eyes looking toward your navel.

10. Inhaling, uncurl your spine, vertebra for vertebra until you reach an upright position, then reach your extended arms up sideways (see inserts) to touch palm to palm overhead. Eyes look up to your hands.

11. Exhaling, lower your arms down sideways, reversing the path taken in step 2 and returning to step 1. Repeat three to 12 times.

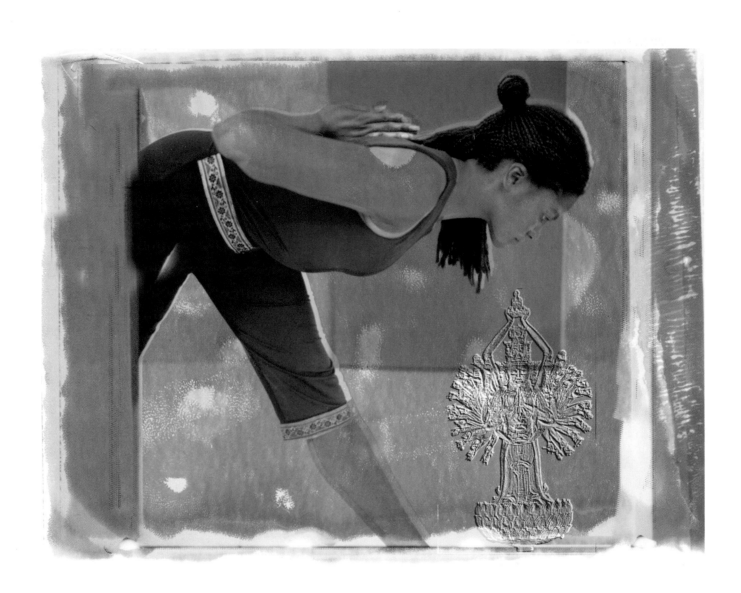

CHAPTER 5

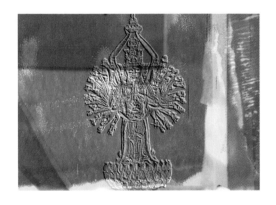

THE POSTURES

The chakras, the body's energy centres

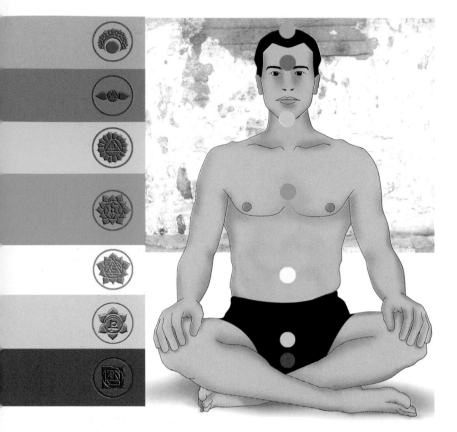

Chakra 6 Ajna (third eye or brow chakra). Colour: indigo. Element: ether. Endocrine system: hypothalamus and pituitary glands. Vital organ: the brain. General function: cognition. Related to wisdom and awareness of the mind.

Chakra 5 Visuddha (throat chakra). Colour: blue. Element: ether. Endocrine system: thyroid and parathyroid, related to the larynx and pharynx. General function: metabolism. Related to communication directed towards others and the self as in the communication between the head and the heart.

Chakra 4 Anahata (heart chakra). Colour: green. Element: air. Endocrine system: thymus gland. Vital organs: heart and lungs. General functions: cardiovascular circulation and respiration. Related to compassion and passion.

Chakra 3 Manipura (solar plexus). Colour: yellow. Element: fire. Endocrine system: none; it is instead associated with the largest bundle of nerves, the solar plexus. Vital organ: pancreas, which influences the stomach and liver. General function: the emotions, relating first to the relationship with the self and extending to relationships with others. This centre can also be understood as being related to awareness of self.

Chakra 2 Svadhisthana (navel chakra or Hara). Colour: orange. Element: water. Endocrine system: adrenal glands. Vital organs: kidneys and intestines. General function: digestion, referring to the absorption and assimilation of nutrients. Related to the ability to absorb, assimilate and nourish on a physical as well as a metaphoric level as an attitude towards life and experience. This centre is also the origin of movement.

Chakra 1 Muladhara (base chakra). Colour: red. Element: earth. Endocrine system: Gonads (ovaries and prostate gland). Vital organs: the reproductive organs and the rectum and anus. General functions: reproduction and elimination. Related to the ability to let go or get rid of the unwanted or unnecessary, as well as relating to the source of abundant energy.

Chakras

Energy (prana) is said to flow in the human body through three main channels (nadis) known as Susumna, Pingala and Ida. Susumna runs through the centre of the spinal column. Ida and Pingala start in the nose (Pingala starting from the right nostril and Ida from the left nostril), move up to the crown of the head and then run downward to the base of the spine. They intersect with each other and with the Susumna nadi at seven junctions. These junctions are known as chakras. The chakras have a regulatory effect on the body and are associated with the endocrine system.

Chakra 7 Sahasrara (crown chakra). Colour: purple (violet). This chakra is associated with light or higher consciousness. Element: none. Endocrine system: pineal gland. Vital organ: the brain. General function: related to faith, enlightenment and higher awareness.

A note on breathing while executing the Yoga postures
Breathing is always through the nose unless otherwise specified.
Each breath is to be slow, deep and evenly timed on inhalation and exhalation.

The postures

In Sanskrit, Yoga postures are called 'asanas'. An asana refers to a position assumed by the physical body, in a comfortable, steady and easy manner – these asanas bring about benefits to the body, the mind and the spirit.

On a physical level, asanas give the body a feeling of lightness, health, poise, flexibility and strength.

On an emotional (or mental) level, they offer the mind a state of calmness and clarity.

On the spiritual level, they free up the communication blocks in the subtle body that block our energy centres (chakras). These benefits to the subtle energy centres are achieved mainly through the balancing effect on the endocrine system and the central nervous system, both of which influence the immune system.

The manner in which the postures are assumed is important. Try not to approach them with frowned seriousness or tension-filled effort – rather be gentle and caring, with a hint of a smile on your face (a smile is an instant reliever of facial tension). It is essential that you enjoy your Yoga practice and very soon you will experience the sense of wellbeing that this practice brings.

The use of asanas is viewed as a gateway to the soul, because by freeing the body of the unnecessary tensions accumulated in daily existence and strengthening the functioning of the various systems of the body, we are able to experience the sense of vitality and joy that Yoga practitioners believe is the true nature of the soul.

This empowering and enhanced sense of vitality will help the practitioner approach any of life's situations.

The levels of difficulty in the postures

It is difficult to devise a system that organizes or rates postures according to degree of difficulty, as there are many factors to take into consideration.

So do keep in mind that while there are many viewpoints about difficulty, this handbook has been based on tried-and-tested methods sourced from various approaches to Yoga.

The rating system decided upon serves as a means of grading the different postures according to degree of difficulty.

Each posture is given a star rating from one to four. The simplest postures, suitable for beginners, have one star, while the most advanced postures have three or four stars. The level of difficulty depends on the required flexibility, strength, balance and co-ordination.

You may find that you are stronger or more naturally flexible in one area than in another, so you may find yourself at level one in some postures and level two or three in others.

If you are a beginner...

- Always begin with the one-star postures, until you can hold them comfortably for the length of time suggested. Then, when you are more confident, you will probably wish to attempt levels two and upwards. The same principle applies to progressing from any number to the next.
- If a posture starts at a two-star level or higher, it means that it is not suitable for beginners and should be attempted when you have more experience. Generally in such cases, other postures are suggested that will serve to prepare your body for being able to attain the posture, in time.
  - You do not need to achieve the most advanced version of a posture in order to gain the benefits. Maximum benefits are gained by staying true to your level and practising the postures comfortably at this level.
  - You will find that you improve over time and will be able to progress onto more advanced levels.
- Don't feel disheartened or inferior if physical restrictions such as muscular tightness, limitations in joint mobility or old injuries prevent your body from attaining some of the more advanced versions. Be assured that you are gaining the benefits at your level of comfort – there is no need to feel any kind of physical pain.
- Read all the instructions carefully and thoroughly. It is a good idea to ask someone else to read them to you when you are new to a posture, to spare you from having to concentrate on reading the instructions at the same time as trying out a posture.
- Take care never to bounce in any posture, and always move into and out of postures slowly, and with care.

The posture groups

This chapter includes Western posture variations and simplifications, which are widely taught and recognized in Yoga classes as ways to introduce postures to the beginner, who will not have the flexibility required to execute a posture in its classical form.

The postures are divided into six groups: sitting postures (including forward bends, back bends and spinal twists), standing postures, standing balances, hand balances, inverted postures and rest postures. Pranayama (breathing practices) has a chapter of its own, Chapter 6.

☀ – ☀ ☀ ☀ ☀ = Grading of posture (from beginner to advanced)

Summary: sitting forward bends

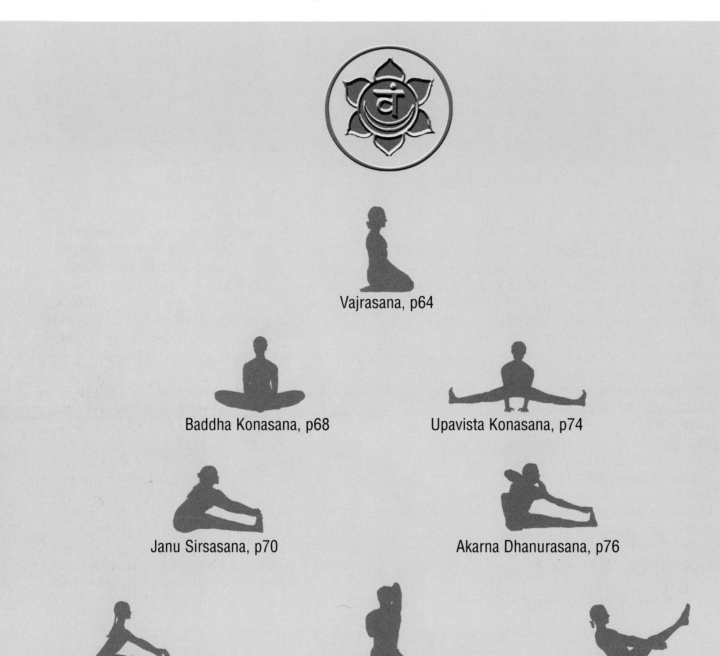

Vajrasana, p64

Baddha Konasana, p68

Upavista Konasana, p74

Janu Sirsasana, p70

Akarna Dhanurasana, p76

Pascimottanasana, p72

Gomukhasana, p66

Paripurna Navasana, p78

SITTING POSTURES
Forward bends

Forward bends in a sitting position generally have a soothing effect on the nervous system, and calm and quieten the mind.

Particularly for beginner Yoga practitioners, sitting forward bends can be easier than standing forward bends, as they do not require the strength and balance that are required for standing postures.

In general, sitting forward bends are good preparations for standing forward bends. They also provide a useful alternative for those who suffer from high blood pressure or a heart condition where it is advisable that the head should never be held below the level of the heart.

Forward bends may influence a number of the energy centres and vital organs at the same time, although, the most prominent centre to benefit is the Svadisthana chakra (navel chakra or second energy centre). This chakra relates to the kidneys and adrenal glands, so practising the forward bend postures is an effective way to balance and strengthen the functions of these organs.

The kidneys

The kidneys relate to the water element. They are responsible for maintaining a state of balance of liquid in the body, by passing any excess liquids down to the bladder for urination, and to the sweat glands, to the eyes in crying or to the nose through the mucous membranes.

The adrenal glands

The adrenal glands produce adrenaline and noradrenaline, which are associated with the survival instinct and fear. The result is a state of increased arousal and energy, preparing the body for 'fight or flight'. This helps us cope with the short-term crises that threaten our survival or wellbeing.

Fear, flight or fight

Because of the stresses of the modern, competitive and fast-paced lifestyle, most people spend larger periods of time than necessary in the mode of 'fight or flight', associated with the activation of the sympathetic nervous system.

People often find it difficult to relax or find the mental clarity that a state of calmness has to offer. Relaxation and calmness are associated with the activation of the parasympathetic nervous system, which can be achieved through the practice of forward bends.

Although fear is often regarded as a negative emotion, it is a necessary part of life. Fear can prevent us from being hurt or from endangering our lives through certain activities. We also learn and grow by facing our fears and developing insight, wisdom and courage.

It is only when fears become debilitating that they become negative, such as when fear brings about an accumulation of unnecessary tensions in the body or when it holds us back from change, exploration and adapting to new situations.

Before you begin

- If the upright and the simplest forward bend are both one star, always start with the upright version before moving into the forward bend.
- Forward bend postures can be done before and after backward bends, side bends and twists.

VAJRASANA
The Diamond
वज्रासन

Vajrasana is referred to as the Diamond pose or the Adamantine pose. The word 'Vajra' translates as 'thunderbolt', and for this reason, Vajrasana may also be referred to as the Thunderbolt pose. Another literal meaning comes from the roots 'va' meaning 'to move' and 'ra' meaning 'radiant'. This posture directs or moves the blood supply and subtle energies to the upper body, all the way up to the head. Thus it prepares or 'radiates' the mind for concentration or meditation, and can be used as a posture for meditation.

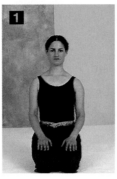
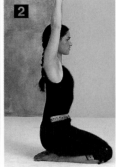
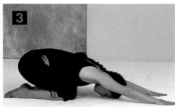

Moving into Supta Vajrasana (in a forward bend)

2. Inhale, then extend your arms overhead, stretching up from the waist. Interlock the fingers, with the palms facing upwards
3. Exhale. Reach forward until the hands touch the ground. Your palms are placed down with the fingers extended away from you. Your forehead rests on the ground and your arms, waist and chest extend forwards.

Upright version ☼

1. Kneel with your legs together and toes pointing out behind you, then sit back on your heels. The big toes touch and the heels are apart, while the spine is extended through the neck. It is important that you feel the length of the spine and neck throughout. Your chin is slightly lowered so that your neck is held in line with the rest of your spine – this will help keep your back straight. Place your hands on your thighs, palms down, just above your knees. Make sure your head and eyes look straight ahead.

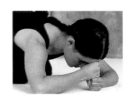

If you have high blood pressure or a heart condition, place your head on two fists or on a cushion in the forward bend so that your head and neck are not below your heart.

Timing: This position can be held for long periods, even half an hour or more as your body gets used to it. You can use the upright posture while carrying out exercises for the neck, eyes, shoulders and arms, and you can use it for meditation. Hold for four to eight breaths before moving into Supta Vajrasana.

Benefits

Supta Vajrasana, Virasana and Mandukasana:

- Restrict blood flow to the legs, thus directing the blood flow to the upper half of the body, nourishing the internal organs.
- Assist digestion, and are all among the few postures that can be practised directly after a meal, to relieve the feeling of fullness.
- Help get rid of flatulence.
- improves the flexibility of the knees.
- Strengthen and stretch the muscles and nerves in the legs and thighs.
- Help relieve sciatica.
- Help to improve flat feet, as these postures help to stretch out the front of the ankle and foot to encourage the development of the arch and instep.

Added benefits of forward bends
- They stretch out the spinal column, relieving tension.
- They give a gentle massage to the abdominal organs, which is how they aid digestion.
- They stretch the lower back, benefiting the kidneys and adrenal glands.
- They calm the nervous system.
- They improve blood circulation to the face and scalp, which can be helpful in preventing wrinkles.

Added benefits of the dynamic version
- It strengthens and tones the abdominal and back muscles.
- Keeps the spine elastic.

Added benefit of Mandukasana
- It stretches the inner thighs.
- It increases flexibility in the hips.

Dynamic version ☀☀

1. Start in Vajrasana and follow the instructions for moving into Supta Vajrasana.
2–3. After exhaling into Supta Vajrasana, inhale reversing the pathway, while rounding the spine. Uncurl, vertebra for vertebra, keeping arms next to the ears, until you return to an upright sitting position with arms next to ears. Keep hands apart and fingers extended.
4. On exhalation, return to Vajrasana.

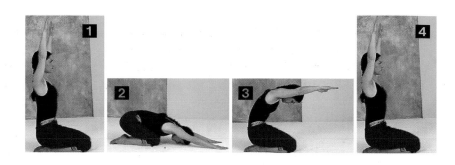

Timing: Repeat three to eight times in a flowing manner, co-ordinating breath with movement.

The following two postures are to be carried out following the same instructions as for Vajrasana and Supta Vajrasana, but with variations in the positioning of the legs.

Virasana ☀☀

A. Place legs as for Vajrasana, then rotate your thighs inward from your hips, so that you are able to sit on the ground between your heels. The insides of your legs rest on the ground, with your lower legs resting on the outer sides of your thighs. In Virasana and Supta Virasana, place your hands on your soles or keep them as for Vajrasana.

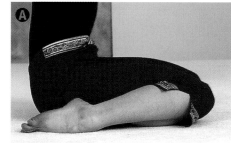
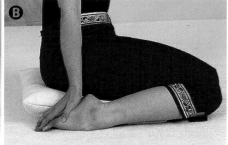

Option

B. Sit on a cushion to ease position of knees.

Mandukasana – the Frog ☀☀

1. Place legs as for Vajrasana, then spread knees wide apart. Keep the big toes touching.
2. Extended version: Shift weight forwards and place your hips on the ground, lying on your front. Rest head on your folded arms.

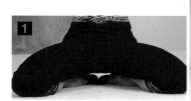
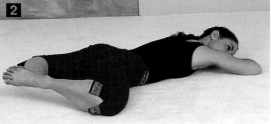

Cautions

- Your knees may take strain, so place one folded blanket or cushion on the inside of your knees, and another to support your hips and soften your seat on your heels.

- If you have varicose veins, it might be best not to attempt this posture – or at least take care while doing it.
- During pregnancy, keep the knees apart in Vajrasana.

GOMUKHASANA
The Cow-face
गोमुखासन

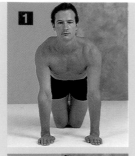

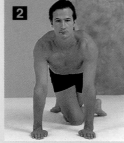

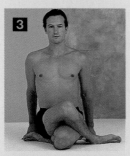

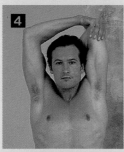

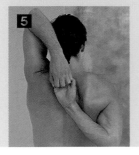

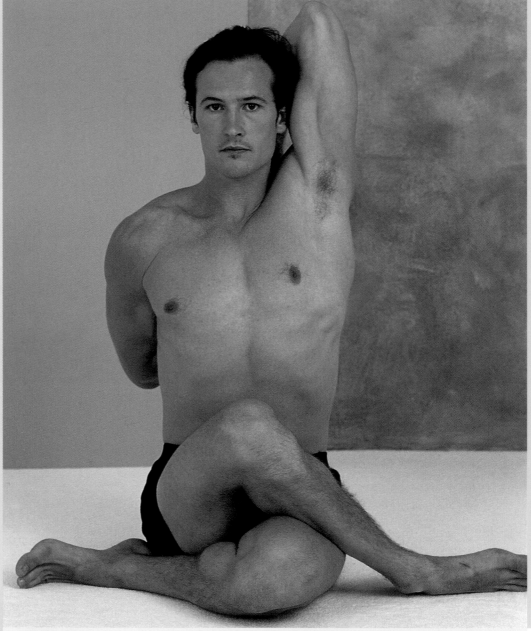

Benefits

- Increases the blood supply to the torso and head area.
- Has an awakening effect on the brain, creating a feeling of lightness in the head and shoulders.
- Expands the chest.
- Loosens the shoulder joints, increasing their flexibility.
- Stretches the thigh muscles and helps to increase the flexibility of the knees.
- Affords mental clarity and benefits the pituitary gland, working mainly on the 6th energy centre (Ajna chakra, or third eye).

Cautions

- Take care to keep your torso centred and balanced throughout, by keeping your spine lengthened. Avoid leaning over to either side while holding the posture.
- If you have a knee, shoulder, elbow or arm problem or injury, stay with the preparatory exercises and even so, only if you can comfortably do so.
- To assist you in achieving the sitting position, you can place a folded blanket or cushion under your hips. If you have varicose veins, use the cross-legged sitting position.

'Go' means cow and 'Mukha' means face. This posture, when viewed from behind, is thought to resemble the face of a cow. 'Go' can also mean 'light'; 'gomukh' in this sense refers to light in or of the head. This refers to the effect of Gomukhasana creating a feeling of lightness in the head area.

Gomukhasana ☀ ☀
The sitting position

1. Kneel with your feet pointing behind you and your hands on the ground in front of you.
2. Place your right leg in front of your left, crossing your legs so that your thighs are touching.
3. Sit down between your heels with lower legs and feet parted. Keep your back upright. Roll your right thigh inward slightly, bringing your feet as close to your hips as you can, so that the position of your legs is tight.

The arm position

4. Start as for the preparatory exercise below. Lower your right arm, bending it at the elbow and raising your hand and forearm behind your back.
5. Clasp your fingers so that you hook your hands together or clasp your hands (palm to palm). In either case, take care that your hands are centred in line with your spine and between your shoulder blades. Clasp hands firmly and keep hands and torso centred. Head and eyes look straight ahead.

Timing: Hold for two to eight breaths.
To recover from the pose, slowly release your hands and arms, reversing the path taken into the posture.
Repeat to the other side, crossing your left leg in front and raising your right arm.

Preparation: ☀
exercises for arms

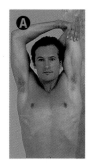

A. Raise your left elbow, placing your left hand on your back, below the nape of your neck and centred between your shoulder blades.
Take hold of your left elbow with your right hand to assist the stretch.
Try to keep your head upright, while easing your left elbow behind your head.

Holding a strap

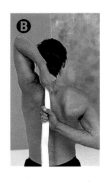

B. Clasp a strap in your left hand and allow it to hang down your spine.
Take hold of the strap and ease your hands as close together as you can, by pulling on the strap.
Hold the posture for three to six breaths, then repeat with your right arm.

Options: the sitting position ☀

A. Sit on a cushion to get used to the position.
B. Sit with legs folded under you.
C. Sit with crossed legs.

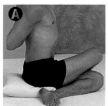
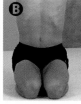
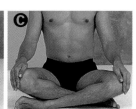

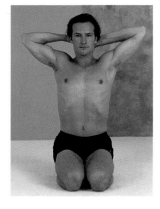

Counter-posture

Sit in Vajrasana or with your legs crossed comfortably. Clasp your fingers (hooking them) behind your neck, with elbows pointing out to the sides. Gently pull your arms away from each other, feeling the stretch across the front of your chest. Take a deep breath, expanding your chest. Hold for three or four breaths.

BADDHA KONASANA
The Butterfly
बद्ध कोणासन

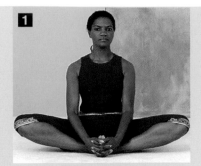

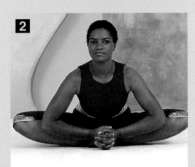

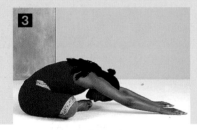

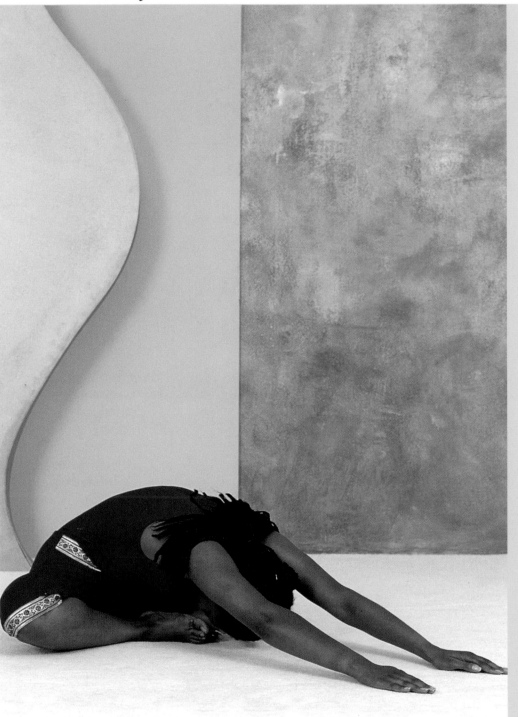

Benefits

- Improves mobility in the hip joint.
- Relieves tension in the sacrum and coccyx.
- Relieves tension in the thighs, knees and ankles.
- Tones the reproductive organs and the bladder.
- Relieves any premenstrual tension and other menstrual problems.
- Helps the pelvic area to prepare for easier childbirth.
- Nourishes the lowest energy centre, the Muladhara, or base chakra (reproductive organs).

The position of the legs in this posture resembles the wings of a butterfly. The posture is also called the Cobbler pose, as it is a position traditionally used by Indian cobblers; it is also known as Badrasana.

Upright position (Baddha Konasana) ☀

1. Sit upright, with knees bent and opened to point to the sides. Your spine is extended. The soles of your feet touch one another and your heels are drawn in close to the body. Keep both knees level and pressed down towards the ground. Hold your feet or ankles in your hands, drawing your heels closer towards you. Keep your chest and shoulders open.

Supta Baddha Konasana ☀ ☀

2. Inhale. Grow taller through spine and head. Exhale. Lean forward from your hips, pushing from the lower part of your spine. Keep your spine extended and your back straight. The chest is open and pushed slightly forward. Hold your feet or ankles close to your body. Pull on them to assist the forward movement. Open your elbows out to the sides. Press your knees toward the ground. Your eye focus is in relation to the position of the head in line with the spine; your eyes are downcast diagonally to the ground in front of you or looking out in front of you.

Extended version ☀ ☀ ☀

3. Stretch your arms out in front of you on the ground, palms down. Lower your forehead towards the ground, keeping your spine as extended as possible.
Caution: If you have a back injury or problem, do not do this extended version.

To recover, inhale, returning slowly to the starting position and gently release your hands and legs.

> **Timing:** Hold for six to eight breaths, concentrating on the hip area and on pressing your knees down towards the ground.
> Note: to enhance the effectiveness of this position, lightly contract the perineum (the sphincter muscles in the pelvic floor).

Preparation: bouncing knees

1–2. Gently bounce your knees up and down, while in Baddha Konasana.

This version prepares the hips and inner thighs to be able to hold the Butterfly with greater ease.

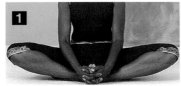 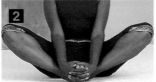

Extra help

A. Sit in the Butterfly facing a wall and place your feet against the wall.
Use your hands next to hips to raise your hips and ease them closer to the wall. Hands remain on the ground for support.
Press knees towards the ground.

This exercise can be used when you find it difficult to hold Baddha Konasana.

Options ☀

A. If you struggle to keep your back straight, sit on a cushion.
B. Hold your ankles in Baddha Konasana.

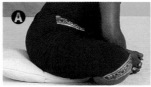 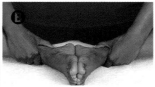

Cautions

• If you have high blood pressure or a heart condition, avoid the version in the full forward bend (remain in the version with the spine extended diagonally forwards).
• When menstruating, do not contract the perineum (pelvic floor muscles).

JANU SIRSASANA
Head to Knee
जानु शीर्षासन

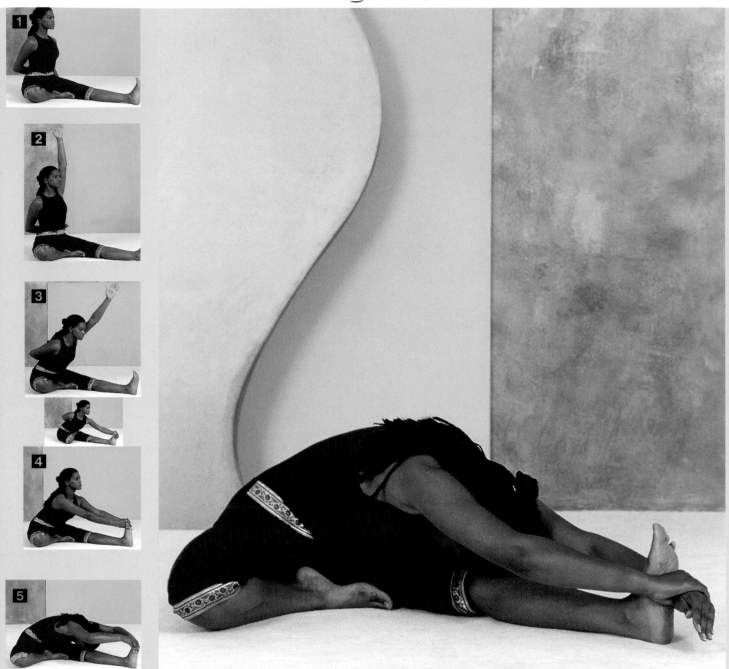

Benefits

- Improves the flexibility of the hamstrings (a group of muscles at the back of the upper leg) and the calf muscles (at the back of the lower leg).
- Strengthens and stretches the back, particularly working on the sacral area of the spine.
- Benefits the kidneys and adrenal glands and generally calms the nervous system.

- Limbers the hips, knees and legs.
- The action of bending forwards gently squeezes and massages the abdominal organs, therefore helping digestion and elimination.
- Asymmetrical poses work to bring balance to the two hemispheres of the brain, as well as to the development of flexibility evenly on both sides of the body. This enhances symmetry and balance in the entire body.

This pose can be used on its own, although it is also a good preparatory pose for Pascimottanasana (p72). Note that Janu Sirsasana is an asymmetrical posture and must therefore be followed by a symmetrical posture, such as Pascimottanasana or the rest posture Apanasana (p149).

Starting position in Dandasana ☀ (the Staff)

1. Sit in Dandasana. Your spine is extended as you hold your your back upright. Arms are at your sides.

   Your legs are extended out in front of you, parallel and together, with the knees locked. Your feet are flexed, reaching forward through the heels.

   Bend your right leg, opening the knee out to the side and pressing it down towards the ground. The left leg remains undisturbed, with the flexed foot pointing upwards.

   Press your right heel into the inner left thigh, as high up on your inner thigh (as close to your groin) as possible.

   Both hips face the front as squarely as possible.

   Bend your right arm and place it behind your lower back. Sit on a cushion if you struggle to keep your lower back straight. Your left arm remains at your side.

Dynamic version (used as a preparation for the static version) ☀

2. Inhaling, raise your left arm forward and up. Place it next to your ear, with your fingers pointing upwards.

3. Exhaling, bend forward from your hips, keeping your spine extended. Your arm remains next to your ear until you reach your maximum forward bend without rounding your spine. Then lower your arm to take hold of your foot or ankle. Keep your head and neck in line with the rest of your spine.

Inhaling, initiate recovery to the upright position at the start of the inhalation by extending your left arm, bringing it once again next to your ear, before sitting upright. This helps to keep your back straight.

Exhaling, lower your arm sideways down to the ground.

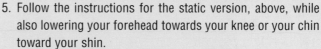

Timing: Repeat this motion three to six times. Then move into the static version.

Static version ☀☀

As for the dynamic version up until the first exhalation to bend forward into Janu Sirsasana. Then:

4. Bring your right hand forward to take hold of the left foot or ankle. Use both hands to assist your forward bend by pulling on your foot or ankle.

   Your eyes look towards your ankle or out in front of you. Hold this position.

   To recover, follow instruction as for the dynamic version.

Janu Sirsasana – Head to Knee pose ☀☀☀

5. Follow the instructions for the static version, above, while also lowering your forehead towards your knee or your chin toward your shin.

   Gently use your arms to assist your forward bend.

   Keep your spine extended as much as possible.

Timing: Hold for four to eight breaths, focusing your attention on keeping your hips square, your abdomen pressed in towards your spine and breathing into your chest area. With each exhalation, try to relax a little further forward. Repeat the movements, this time with your right leg extended.

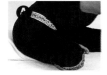

Option ☀

A. If you struggle to keep your lower back straight, sit on a cushion throughout, so that your hips are raised slightly.

Cautions

- If you have a back problem, do not take your head to your knee while holding this posture. Remain in the version with your spine extended and your head raised.

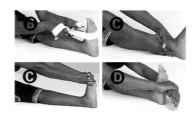

Options for hands

B. Hold a strap slung around your foot..

C. Hold your lower legs, ankles or toes.

D. Hold your left wrist in your right hand, around your foot.

PASCIMOTTANASANA
Sitting Forward Bend
परिचमोत्तानासन

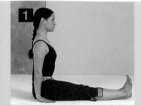
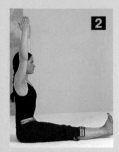
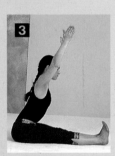
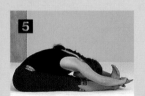
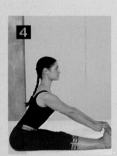

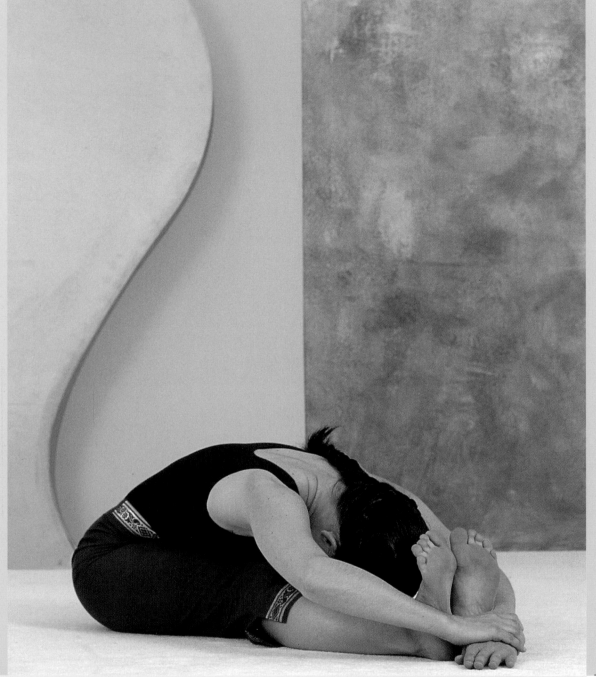

Benefits

- Gives a good stretch to the spine, helping to improve posture and the health of the spinal column, particularly in the sacral region.
- Loosens the hamstrings (the muscles at the back of the upper legs).
- Increases blood flow to the spine, nourishing the nerve networks extending out from the spine.
- Brings a fresh blood supply to the pelvic area, thus benefiting the reproductive organs.

- Influences the adrenal glands, which are located just above and slightly in front of the kidneys. This has a calming influence, as it helps to activate the para-sympathetic nervous system.
- Gives a gentle squeeze and massage to the abdominal organs, helping to tone them.
- It can be helpful in alleviating constipation, as it aids digestion and elimination.
- The dynamic version particularly strengthens the back and abdominal muscles.

'Pascima' literally means 'the west'. The back is considered to be the west side of the body and the front the east. 'Utana' means 'to stretch'. Thus Pascimottanasana refers to stretching the west side of the body (the back), and is sometimes called the 'back-stretching' posture.

Starting position in Dandasana (the Staff) ☀

1. Your spine is extended as your back is held upright. Your head and neck are held in line with your spine and your eyes are looking forward.

   The navel is pressed towards the spine, so that you breathe into your chest area.

   Your shoulders are relaxed and open. Keep your arms at your sides, resting hands or fingers on the floor. Your legs are held parallel and together, at a right angle to the torso and extended out in front of you. Your knees are locked.

   Your feet are flexed, with the toes pointing upwards. Reach forward through your heels.

Dynamic version ☀

2. Start in Dandasana. Inhaling, raise your arms forward and upward, placing them next to your ears. Extend upwards through the fingers.

3. Exhaling, bend forward from the hips, keeping arms next to ears. This helps keep the back straight and the neck aligned.

4. When you can bend forward no further without rounding your spine, lower your arms and place your hands on your shins, ankles or feet. Eyes look toward your ankles or straight out in front of you.

Inhaling, initiate recovery to upright at the start of the inhalation, by extending your arms, bringing them once again next to your ears, which helps to keep your back straight. Reverse the path taken into the forward bend to return to an upright position.

Exhaling, lower your arms sideways to the ground, returning to Dandasana.

Timing: Repeat this motion three to six times. Then move into the static version.

Static version ☀☀

Execute as for the dynamic version, holding after the first exhalation into the forward bend. Maintain the length of your spine and keep legs extended and parallel. Breathe into your chest area, expanding the front and back of your ribcage on inhalation.

Static Full Pascimottanasana ☀☀☀

5. Execute as for static version, lowering your forehead or chin towards your shins. Pull on your feet or ankles with your hands to help increase your forward bend. Hold your elbows out to the sides to avoid straining your shoulders. Relax your neck and head onto or toward your legs.

Timing: Hold for four to eight or up to 16 breaths, focusing your attention on keeping legs stretched, abdomen pressed in toward the spine and the spine extended. With each exhalation, feel that you can relax a little further forward. Your spine should feel stretched and relaxed. To recover, follow instructions as for the dynamic version.

Option ☀

A. If you struggle to keep your lower back straight, sit on a cushion throughout so that your hips are raised slightly.

Options for hands

B. Hold a strap slung around your foot.
C. Hold your lower legs, ankles or big toes.
D. Hold your left wrist in your right hand, wrapped around your feet.

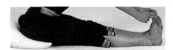

Cautions

• If your back or legs are tight, or if you have a back injury, bend your knees slightly, keeping your back straight as you bend forward. Gradually work towards straightening your legs.

• If you have a back problem or high blood pressure, do not take your head to your knee while holding this pose. Remain with your spine extended diagonally.

• If you are pregnant, part your legs to make space for your abdomen in the forward bend.

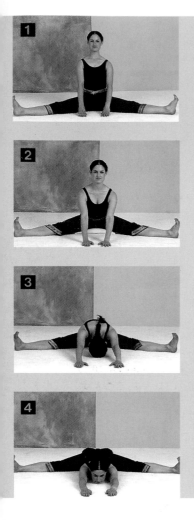

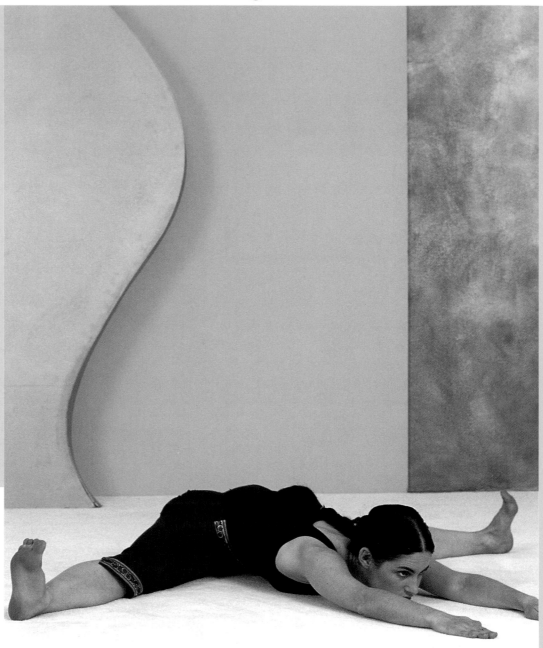

Benefits

- Increases flexibility of the inner thighs.
- Stretches and strengthens the back.
- Improves mobility in the hip joint.
- Benefits the reproductive organs.
- The twisted version gives a lateral extension to the torso.

Cautions

- If you have high blood pressure or a heart condition, either remain in the position with your spine extended at a diagonal to your legs, or place your elbows on the ground in the forward bend, so that your head always remains above the level of your heart.

'Upavista' means 'seated' and 'kona' means 'angle'. This refers to a sitting position where the torso is held at an angle to the legs, with the legs also forming an angle to each other as they are opened out to the sides. The English name 'Straddle' is often used to describe this posture.

Upavista Konasana ☀

1. Sit in Dandasana (p73). Spread your legs as far apart as you can, keeping your feet flexed.
2. Place your hands on the ground in front of you. Inhaling, grow taller through your spine.
3. Exhaling, lean forward from your hips, keeping your spine extended and your head and neck in line with your spine. Your eyes are downcast relative to the position of your head. Walk your hands forward on the ground as you

lean forward. Take care to keep your weight evenly distributed on both buttocks.

Extended version ☀ ☀ ☀

4. Execute as for Upavista Konasana, walking your hands out in front of you, so that you bring your chest and head closer to the ground. Aim to place on the ground either your elbows or the crown of your head, or your chest and chin.

Timing: Hold for four to 16 breaths. The focus of attention is on the stretch of your inner thighs and on keeping your legs extended through your heels. Also focus on rotating your inner thighs outward, so that your feet point upwards throughout. To recover, inhale, reversing the path taken into the posture.

Dynamic Parsva Upavista Konasana (Sideways Straddle) ☀ ☀

Start in Dandasana with the legs spread apart.

1–2. Inhaling, reach your arms up next to your ears and turn your upper body, from the waist, to face your right leg.
3. Exhaling, bend forward over your right leg, keeping spine extended and arms next to your ears. When you can bend no further without rounding your spine, place your hands on your right ankle or foot. Gently pull on the ankle or foot to assist (holding your elbows to the sides so that your shoulders don't strain).

Keep your left leg extended and your weight on both buttocks. Hold for three to six breaths.

4. Inhaling, bring your arms next to the ears and return to the centred, upright position, with your spine extended throughout the movement.
5. Turn your upper body to the left.
6. Exhaling, repeat forward bend to the left. Inhaling, recover to the upright, centred position.

Timing: Repeat three to six times.

After doing Parsva Upavista Konasana, move into Upavista Konasana (with forward bend to the centre), as a counter-posture to restore symmetry to the body.

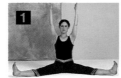 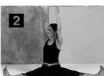 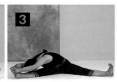 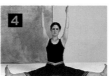 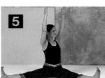 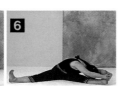

Options for holding Upavista Konasana

A. Place your elbows on the ground.
B. Place the crown of your head on the ground.
C. Place your cheek on the ground with your head turned sideways and arms stretched out to the sides or holding your big toes.

Options ☀

A. Sit on a cushion if you find yourself struggling to keep your back straight.
B. If your inner thighs or lower back are tight, bend your knees slightly. Work toward straightening your legs.

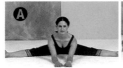 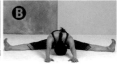 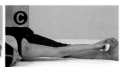 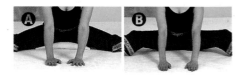

AKARNA DHANURASANA
The Shooting Bow
आकर्ण धनुरासन

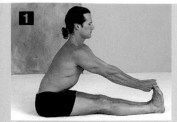

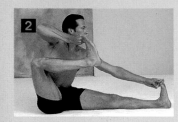

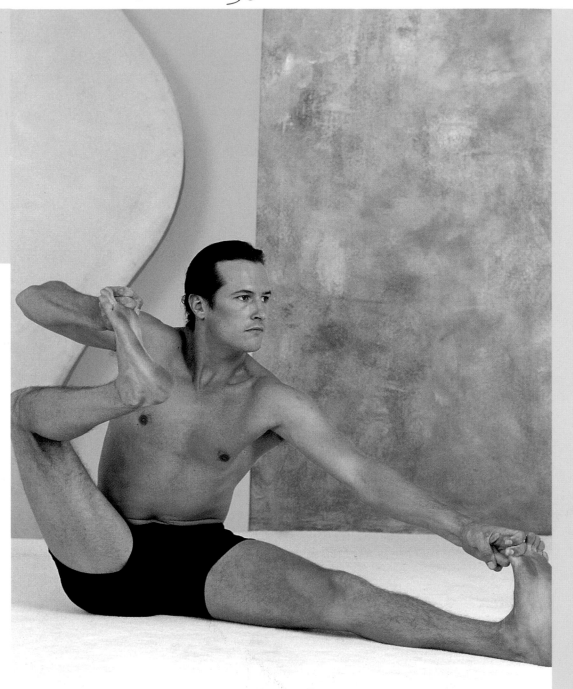

Benefits

- Increases flexibility in the legs and hips.
- Strengthens and stretches the feet and ankles, as well as the arms and hands.
- Focuses the mind and its attention.
- Stretches and strengthens the back.
- Can alleviate rheumatism in the legs and sciatica.
- Gives a squeeze to the abdomen, thus aiding digestion and elimination.

Cautions

- Be careful not to turn your head while holding Akarna Dhanurasana.
- If you have a spinal injury or problem, do not attempt this posture.

The prefix 'a' means 'near to' or 'towards', 'karna' means 'ear' and 'dhani' means 'bow'. Thus Akarna Dhanurasana refers to a posture that draws the foot towards the ear as if it were a bow-string of an archer preparing to shoot an arrow. The other hand holds the other foot in place as if it were the stick of the bow; eyes are focused ahead as if taking aim at a target. Practise Pascimottanasana and Upavista Konasana before attempting Akarna Dhanurasana.

Akarna Dhanurasana ☀ ☀ ☀

1. Start in Dandasana (p73)
   Reach forward, keeping your back straight, and take hold of your big toes (right toe in right hand, left in left).
   Keep head and neck in line with the rest of your spine with the focus of the eyes straight out in front of you.
   Inhaling, extend through the spine.
2. Exhaling, draw your right leg up, bending the knee out to the side. Bring your foot as close as you can to your ear, with your right elbow raised. Your torso will rotate to the right. Take care to keep your chest up and your head and

eyes looking forward (as if taking aim at a target in front of you) in line with your left leg that remains extended on the ground, with your foot flexed and your left hand holding the big toe.
Keep your weight evenly distributed on both buttocks.

After doing the posture on both sides, hold the symmetrical forward bend, or move into Supta Baddha Konasana (p69) and hold for four to six breaths to restore symmetry to the body.

Timing: Hold for two to six breaths. Focus your attention on the pull in two directions, between your hands and feet.
To recover, on an inhalation reverse the path taken into the position, returning to the forward bend holding the big toes.
Hold for two to three breaths, then repeat using the left leg. Hold the posture for an equal length of time on both sides.
Repeat two or three times, alternating legs and moving into the extended version on the second or third repetition.

Preparation: leg rocking ☀ ☀

1. Start in a comfortable, cross-legged sitting position, with spine extended and right leg on top of left. Lift your right leg up toward your chest with both hands, keeping your knee open to the side. Cradle your lower leg by placing the right foot in the crook of the left elbow and the right knee in the crook of the right elbow, arms wrapped around the front of the lower leg. Interlock your fingers and hug your leg close in to your chest, as if cradling a baby.
2. Gently rock your leg from side to side or hold for two to six breaths. Aim to keep your back as straight as you can.
   To recover, on an exhalation return your right leg to the starting position. Rest for a breath or two, then repeat pose on the opposite side .
   To restore symmetry after doing both sides, place the soles of your feet together and bend forward over your legs (as for Supta Baddha Konasana, p69).

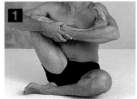
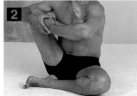

Preparation: leg raises ☀ ☀

1. Lie on your back on the ground with legs parallel and extended, feet flexed and arms at your sides.
2–3. Bend your left leg, taking hold of the outside of your left foot in your left hand. Ease your left knee down towards your left armpit. Raise your lower leg to a vertical position with your sole facing upward. Keep your right leg extended and the back of your right hip in contact with the ground.
   Hold for three to six breaths, then repeat with the right leg.

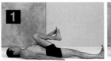
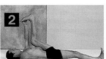
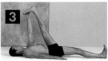

Extended version ☀ ☀ ☀ ☀

Start as for Akarna Dhanurasana. Extend your right leg upwards, aiming to straighten your leg.
To recover, on an inhalation, reverse the path taken into the posture, and repeat with the other leg.

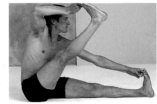

PARIPURNA NAVASANA
The Boat
नावासन नावासन

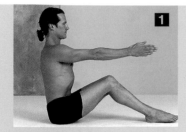

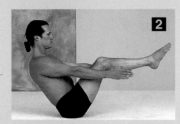

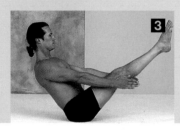

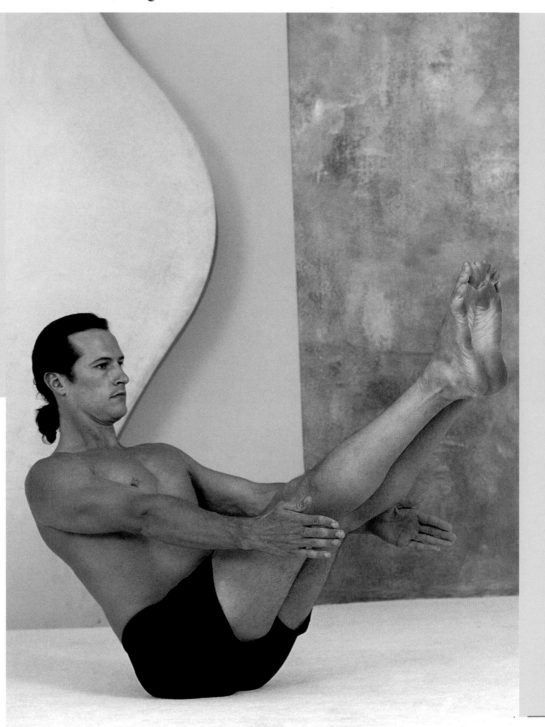

Benefits

- Strengthens and tones the muscles of the abdomen, the legs and the back.
- Improves balance.
- Tones the intestines.
- Limbers the legs and hips.

Cautions

- Take care not to hold your breath while balancing.
- If you are straining while doing this posture, rather hold the balance for a shorter period of time and repeat two or three times. You can also rest for a few recovery breaths in between.

'Paripurna' means 'complete' or 'entire', while 'navasana' means 'a boat'. Paripurna Navasana refers to a balancing posture that resembles a boat, where the balance is held on the buttocks, with the body forming a 'V' shape. It requires strength in the back and abdominal muscles. When the 'V'-shape is wider and the torso and legs are held closer to the ground, this posture is called Ardha Navasana.

Paripurna Navasana ☀ ☀

1. Sit upright with legs together, knees bent and the soles of the feet on the ground. The arms are extended, with the hands and fingers pointing forward and arms parallel to the ground.
2. Lean backwards, balancing your weight by raising your lower legs off the ground. Extend your feet. Take care to keep your spine extended, lifting from your lower spine. The head and neck are held in line with your spine.
Hold in this position or move on to the full posture.
3. Extend your legs, so that your body forms a 'V' shape, with your feet pointed.

Timing: Hold for three to eight breaths. Focus your attention on feeling your spine and legs extending diagonally away from each other, and reach forwards with your arms.

Ardha Navasana ☀ ☀

1. Start in Dandasana (p75). Interlock your fingers behind your head, with the elbows held slightly in on either side of your head.
2. On an exhalation lean backwards, lowering your back towards the ground and raising your extended legs a small distance off the ground.
Balance in this position, looking towards your feet.
Recover by returning to the sitting position and rest for a few recovery breaths in Savasana (p148). This balance can be repeated two or three times in order to strengthen your back and abdominal muscles.

Ubhaya Padangusthasana ☀ ☀ ☀

A. Start in Paripurna Navasana. Take hold of your big toes and gently bring your legs closer in toward your face. Keep your legs extended, held together and parallel, and make sure your spine is extended.

Variation: with legs apart ☀ ☀ ☀

B. Start in Ubhaya Padangusthasana, then open your legs out to the sides, with the help of your arms. Push forwards in your chest and lower back to help your balance. This balance can also be started from Baddha Konasana (p68). Take hold of your big toes in this position and lean back as you extend one leg at a time.

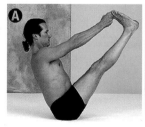

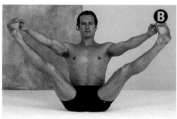

Summary: back bends

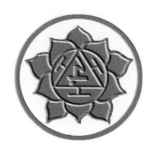

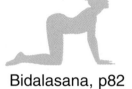

Bidalasana, p82

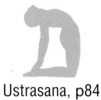

Ustrasana, p84

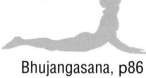

Bhujangasana, p86

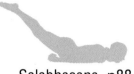

Salabhasana, p88

Dhanurasana, p90

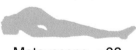

Matsyasana, p92

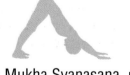

Adho Mukha Svanasana, p94

Urdhva Dhanurasana, p96

SITTING POSTURES
Back bends

Back bends generally require strength, while the forward bends require flexibility. At the same time, back bends are a good way in which to strengthen and tone the body, particularly the muscles of the back, legs and buttocks. If you feel that you lack the initial strength to begin back bends, practise a one-star level standing posture such as Virabhadrasana.

The spine and the nervous system

Back bends increase flexibility of the spinal column, helping to improve posture and keeping the spine elastic. They also benefit the nervous system by increasing the blood supply to the spinal area and to the nerves that extend out from the spinal cord.

Digestion and breathing

Back bends stretch the abdominal area and greatly assist digestion as they tone the often weak abdominal muscles and digestive organs.

They also expand and open the chest area and enhance flexibility in the shoulders, which helps to facilitate chest expansion. This encourages deeper breathing, benefiting the respiratory system and helping to improve posture. While holding the body in a back bend, the mind is brought to a state of passive stillness.

The pancreas and the spleen

Back bends influence a number of the energy centres. Whenever the neck is stretched backwards or the chin raised, for example, the Visuddha chakra, the energy centre in the throat area, is influenced.

In full back bends, all the chakras are influenced. However, the chakra that is most influenced, and therefore receives the most benefit, is the Manipura chakra, the third energy centre, which relates to the solar plexus area.

This chakra is also related to the pancreas, which exerts a chemical influence on the stomach and the liver, as well as to the spleen. On an energetic level, all these organs are seen to support one another.

The pancreas is involved in regulating the body's sugar levels by producing insulin. If the insulin levels reduce, diabetes can be the result, and the muscles are no longer able to make efficient use of glucose. The function of the spleen is to distinguish between pure and impure ingested food.

These physical functions and their related chakras are reflected in our emotions too. For example, it is essential that we are able to distinguish between what is valuable and what is not. When the energy of the spleen becomes blocked, the negative emotions that result are associated with obsessive thought, excessive worrying and a feeling of being 'stuck'. In this way, the spleen influences our ability to make decisions and to move forward in life. (This view ties in with the solar plexus, since worrying is often felt as a knot of tension in the area between the navel and the ribcage, the region of the solar plexus.)

The pancreas is associated with the way we handle change in our lives. This energy relates to thought and the ability to reflect on things and turn them over in our minds.

Before you begin

- Never do a spinal twist directly before or after a back bend, as it can be dangerous to the spine.
- If you do not follow a back bend by a forward bend, it could lead to discomfort.
- Make sure you are well warmed up, particularly in your back and shoulders, before doing back bends.
- If you have a spinal injury or lower-back problem, support the back bend by tightening your buttock muscles and working to improve flexibility in your upper and middle back. With caution, back bends can strengthen the back.

BIDALASANA
The Cat Stretch

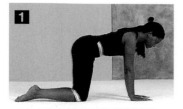

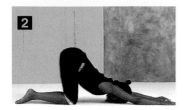

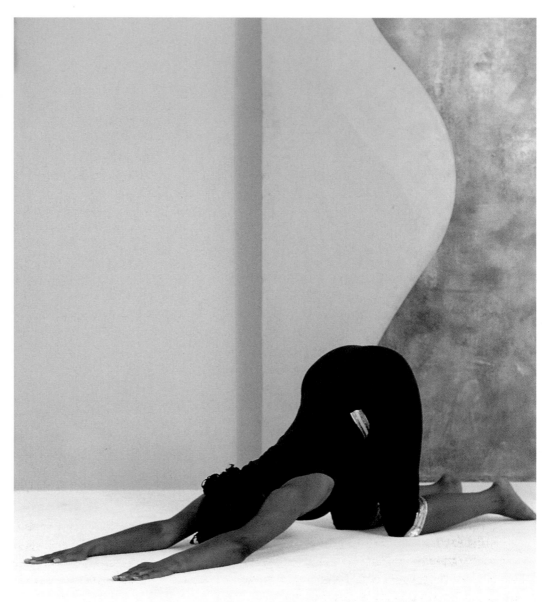

Benefits

- Relaxes the back, particularly the lower spine.
- Can relieve backache and fatigue.
- The Full Cat Stretch relieves tension in the lower back and aligns the vertebrae in the area.
- Improves blood flow to the spine and spinal nerves.
- Opens the chest area.
- Helpful for asthma and other respiratory disorders.
- Strengthens, tones and stretches the abdominal and back muscles, massaging the abdominal organs.
- Improves spinal flexibility.
- Helpful for constipation.
- Helpful for diabetes.
- Very beneficial during pregnancy.

Cautions

- Keep your shoulders down and your neck extended.
- If you have a neck injury or problem, use your neck with care, involving it as little as possible in the motion while hollowing and rounding your spine.

This posture resembles a cat stretching and may also be referred to as Chakravakasana or Utthitha Kummerasana. It offers a gentle and effective way to warm up and stretch the back and abdominal muscles. Bidalasana is a good warm-up for the spine to prepare for back bends.

Full Cat Stretch ☀☀

1. Start on your hands and knees.
2. Walk your hands forward until your forehead can be placed on the ground. Keep your hips raised, so that your thighs remain at right angles to the ground. Reach forwards and out through your chest, arms and fingertips.

Timing: Hold for three to eight breaths or for as long as you wish, as it can be a very comfortable position and very relieving for lower-back tension. To recover, sit back on your heels and rest in the Child's pose (p149) for a few recovery breaths.

Preparation
Cat Stretch on all fours ☀

1. Start on all fours with knees under hips and hands under shoulders. Fingers point forward and head and neck are held in line with the rest of your spine, so that your eyes look to the ground between your hands.
2. Inhaling, hollow your back so that your navel lowers towards the ground. Your chest expands as your back arches and head and chin are raised so that the front of your neck is stretched. Your tailbone is raised to increase the arch in your lower back. Keep your shoulders pressing down, so that your neck is long.
3. While exhaling, round your spine, initiating the movement at the navel, bringing your chin to your chest.
   Repeat, alternating the hollowing and rounding of your spine, three to six times, co-ordinating breath with movement. This mobilizes the back and abdominal muscles and incorporates a forward and a back bend.
   To increase the effectiveness of this pose, contract the pelvic floor throughout (unless menstruating).

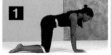 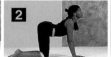 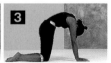

Extended Cat Stretch ☀☀☀

A. Execute as for the Full Cat Stretch, reaching further forward to place your chin and chest on the ground.

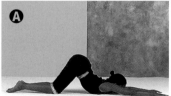

Cat Stretch: with legs ☀☀

Perform this posture as for the Cat Stretch on all fours, but include leg movements:

1. Inhaling, hollow your spine, while raising your right leg so that it extends straight out behind you. Your foot can be pointed or flexed.
2. Exhaling, round your spine, while bending your right leg, bringing your knee in toward your forehead.

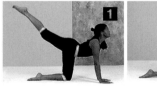 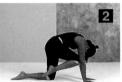

Alternate these two movements, as for the previous exercise, then return to all fours and repeat using your left leg. You can hold the back bend after the inhalation for three to six breaths, before rounding your spine or returning to all fours.

Cat Stretch including leg and arm movements ☀☀☀

1. Inhaling, reach forward with the opposite arm (fingers pointed) to your raised leg.
2. Exhaling, curl your elbow towards your incoming knee.
   This can also be done using the same arm as your working leg, bringing your elbow to your side on exhalation.

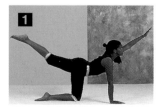 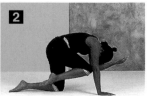

USTRASANA
The Camel
अष्ट्रासन

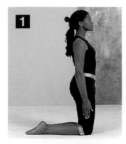

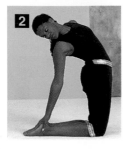

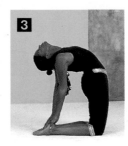

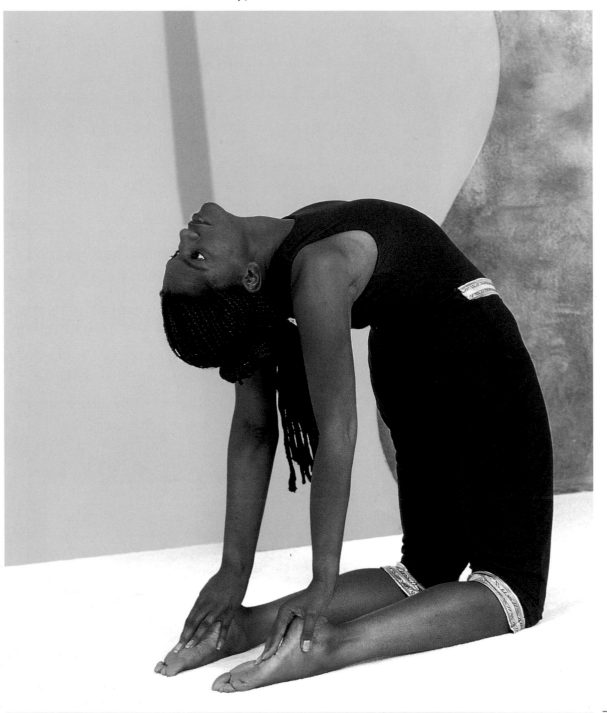

Benefits

- Increases mobility in the spine and shoulders.
- Increases the flexibility of the spine.
- Nourishes and revitalizes the spinal nerves with a fresh blood supply.
- Improves posture.
- Stretches the abdomen, helping to reduce fat.
- Expands the chest and helps to counter a hunched back and rounded shoulders.
- Opens the throat area and relaxes the neck.
- It is helpful for asthma, bronchitis and other respiratory complaints.
- It is beneficial during pregnancy (although it must be done with caution).

'Ustra' means 'camel' in Sanskrit. It also has been translated as meaning 'that which casts light on the mind' and 'that which can help to release knowledge when there is a quest for it'. This is where there is a connection with the camel: camels can survive in the desert by storing water and being able to tap into their store of nourishment when they need it. Likewise, we store knowledge in our minds, which we can use to nourish our spirits if we learn how to tap into it. The Camel revitalizes the mind.

The Half Camel ☀ ☀

1. Start sitting up on your knees, with legs together and feet pointing out behind you.
2. Inhaling, bend backwards, placing your right hand on your right heel, with left hand at your side. Hold for three or four breaths. To recover, exhale and return to the upright position and repeat on the other side, or continue to the full posture.

Ustrasana (the Camel) ☀ ☀ ☀

3. Complete steps 1 and 2, then place both hands on your heels. Rotate your shoulders and arms outward in the position to open your chest and shoulders.
Relax your head backwards, so that the front of your neck is stretched out.

Timing: Hold for three to eight breaths. Recover as for the Half Camel.

To recover from the Camel

1–4. From the Camel, move into the Half Camel, then slowly straighten your spine while rolling your head and upper body to the side and then forwards. Uncurl your spine to the upright position.

Preparation ☀

1. Sit upright on your knees, with your legs together or slightly apart. Place your hands above your buttocks, on your lower back, with elbows pulled behind you, to open your chest.
2. Inhaling, bend your upper spine backwards, while pushing forwards in your hips as you aim to keep your thighs vertical. Raise your head and chin upwards, stretching the front of your neck.

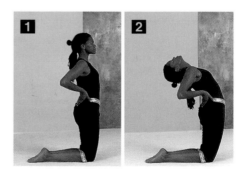

Exhaling, return to the upright position using the strength of your abdominal muscles to initiate the motion.
Repeat three to six times to warm up the spine and strengthen the abdominal muscles. Keep your neck extended and shoulders pressed down throughout.

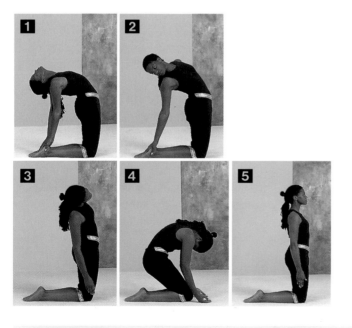

Cautions

• If you have a spinal injury or a neck problem, keep your head upright throughout, in order to avoid involving your neck in the back bend.

BHUJANGASANA
The Cobra
मुजगासन

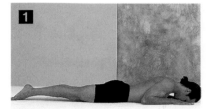

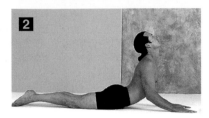

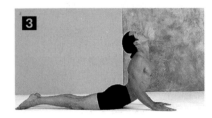

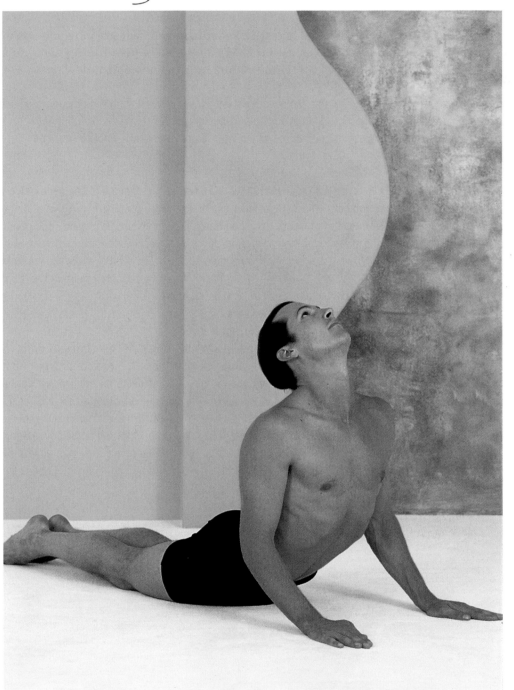

Benefits

- Strengthens the back muscles.
- Increases flexibility and mobility of the spine and vertebrae, particularly in the upper and middle back.
- Increases blood circulation to the spine and nerves.
- Stretches and strengthens neck and shoulder muscles.
- Expands the chest and frees the throat area.

- Strengthens and tones abdominal muscles and organs.
- Helps digestion and can alleviate flatulence.
- Strengthens the function of and revitalizes the kidneys and adrenal glands.
- Increases blood flow to the pelvic area, nourishing the organs (particularly beneficial when followed by the Locust, p88).

In Sanskrit, 'Dhanura' means 'bow'. Dhanurasana is a posture that resembles an archer's bow. Prepare for this posture with Bhujangasana (p86) and Salabhasana (p88) to build the strength and flexibility required for Dhanurasana.

Preparation: the dynamic version ☀ ☀

1. Lie flat on your abdomen, with forehead on the ground and arms straight and held in at your sides, palms up. Keep your legs together and feet extended throughout.
2. Inhaling, stretch your arms backwards, raising them off the ground, as you raise your chest, shoulders, head and legs. The weight of your body rests on your abdomen and hips. Keep your shoulders pressed down and your neck extended; your eyes look straight out in front of you. Exhaling, relax back to the starting position. Repeat three to six times to build strength for the full posture.

Dhanurasana: the Bow ☀ ☀ ☀

Hold the position after inhaling into Dhanurasana, bending your lower legs and taking hold of your feet or ankles.

Timing for static version: Hold for three to eight breaths. Focus your attention on the stretching of the front of your body. To recover, on an exhalation return to the relaxed starting position, lying on your abdomen with your forehead on the ground or turn your head sideways. Hold for a few recovery breaths.

Preparation: the Half Bow ☀ ☀

1. Lie flat on your abdomen, with your elbows placed under your shoulders and palms on the ground. The weight of your upper body rests on your elbows.
2. Inhaling, bend your right knee and reach backwards with your right arm to take hold of your right ankle with your right hand.
3. Raise your right knee off the ground. Hold this position for three to six breaths to prepare your body for the Full Bow.

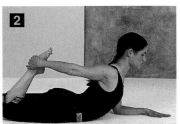
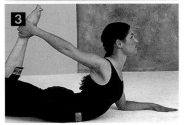

Options for arms

A. Bend your elbows and place your hands together under your forehead.
B. Reach your arms forward and hold them next to your ears.

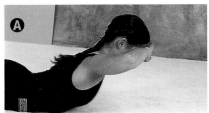
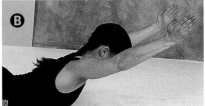

Cautions

- Be well practised in the Cobra and the Locust before attempting the Bow.
- Take care if you have a past spinal injury, perhaps staying with simple versions.
- Make sure you keep your heels as far away from your buttocks as possible.
- Keep head and eyes looking straight ahead if you have a neck problem or past injury.
- Take care not to strain in this position.

MATSYASANA
The Fish
मत्स्यासन

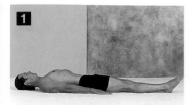

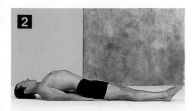

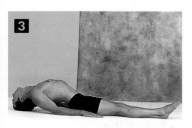

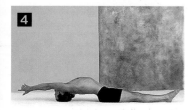

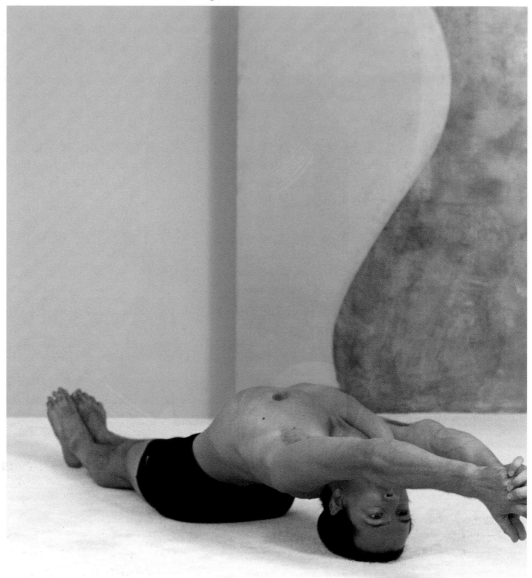

Benefits

- Expands the chest and encourages deeper breathing.
- Opens and stretches the throat area also encouraging deeper breathing.
- Benefits the thyroid and parathyroid glands in the neck, which are the regulators of metabolism.
- Benefits the respiratory system, and is therefore helpful for asthma and bronchitis.
- Relieves tension in the upper back.

- Strengthens the back and nourishes the spinal nerves.
- Increases blood supply to the head area, nourishing the pituitary and the pineal gland where the top of the head is placed on the ground.
- Increases mobility in the pelvic area and tones the organs in this region.
- Offers relief from piles.
- Helps digestion and elimination.
- Helpful for menstrual disorders.

One reason for this posture's name is that, when viewed from above, the body resembles a fish. Another reason is that in this position you will be able to float well in water. Matsyasana – the Fish can be used as a counter-posture after the Shoulder Stand (p138) and the Plough (p140).

Moving into the Fish ☀

1. Lie flat on your back, with legs straight and held together. Rotate legs inward from hips, so that they are parallel. Check that your body is lying in a straight line. Place your hands, palms down, at your sides, next to your thighs.

2. Inhaling, arch your back, raising your torso off the ground with your chest pushing upwards, as if starting to sit up. Press down on your elbows to assist you in attaining the position. Your neck and head remain on the ground.
   Once you are in the position, rest the weight of your body on your elbows for support, keeping elbows in at your sides to open your chest.
   Hold in this position or move into the full posture.

The Fish ☀☀

1–2. Follow the instructions for moving into the posture.

3. Inhaling, raise your head, lightly placing the crown of your head on the ground. To do this, tilt your neck and chin backwards, so that the front of your neck and throat are open and stretched. Keep your elbows in at your sides, so that your chest is also open.
   Hold in this position or move on to the extended version.

The Fish: extended version ☀☀☀

4. Stretch your arms above your head, joining your hands in the Prayer pose (clasp your hands with your index fingers pointing forward).

Timing: Hold for two to eight breaths, focusing your attention on the opening across your chest and the gentle squeeze in your back. If you are using Matsyasana as a counter-posture to the Shoulder Stand or Plough, remain in Matsyasana for a third of the time that you held the Shoulder Stand or Plough. To recover, exhale reversing the path taken into the position, returning to the starting position of lying flat on the ground. Take a few recovery breaths and then move into a simple forward bend or a rest pose, such as the Child's pose (p149).

Preparation: the Fish as a rest pose ☀

A&B. Lie over a cushion or a folded blanket, placing it under the middle of your back, so that your chest is expanded and your back arched over the cushion or blanket. Arms rest on the ground either at shoulder height at your sides or reaching upward, alongside your head. This exercise helps increase flexibility in the back in a relaxed way. It must be followed by a forward bend.

Option: sitting on your hands ☀☀

1. Place hands, with palms down, underneath your buttocks, so that you are sitting on them, with index fingers touching underneath you.

2. Keep your elbows in at your sides and press down in your elbows to assist your moving into the position.
   This version provides a stable support for your body while your are holding Matsyasana.

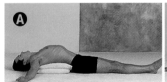
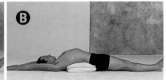
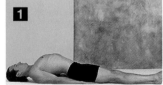
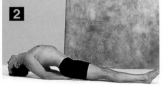

Cautions

• Place your weight lightly on the top of your head in the full posture by resting your weight on your elbows for strong support.

• Do not bend your neck too far backwards in the full posture, as this will strain your neck vertebrae.

• If you have a neck problem, stay with steps 1–2 (p92) and keep your neck and head on the ground.

ADHO MUKHA SVANASANA
Downward-facing Dog Stretch
अधो मुख श्वानासन

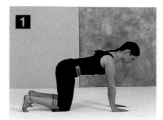

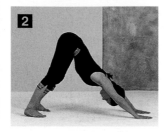

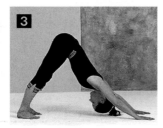

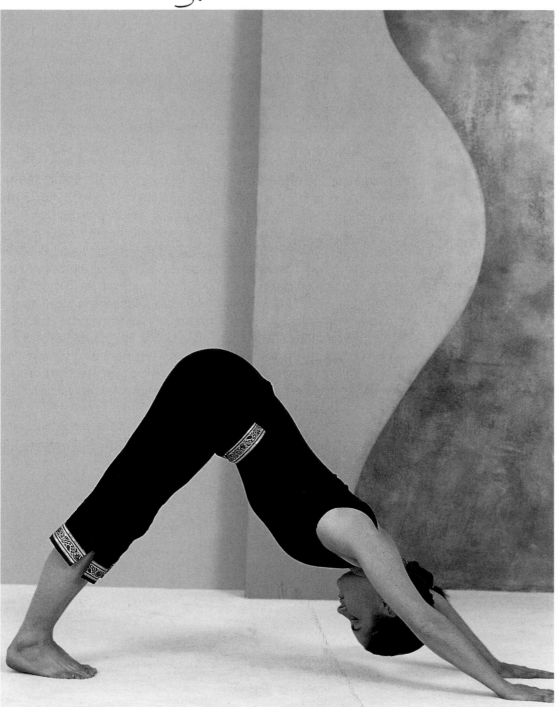

Benefits

- Stretches and relaxes the spine.
- Increases the flexibility of the spine, hamstrings, calf muscles and shoulders.
- Nourishes the brain with an increased blood supply.
- Improves concentration.
- Helpful for insomnia.
- Expands the chest.
- Gives the heart and digestive system a break in the anti-gravity position.
- Gives the abdominal organs a gentle massage.
- Helpful for anaemia.

'Adho Mukha' means 'downward facing', while 'svana' means a dog. This posture imitates a dog stretching. The Downward-facing Dog Stretch is an inverted posture as well as a forward bend. When the back can be arched (as is the aim) while holding the Downward-facing Dog Stretch, the back bend is evident.

Preparation: dynamic version ☀

1. Kneel on all fours with legs together or apart with knees under hips and hands under shoulders (or slightly in front of them). The fingers point forward and toes are curled under, with feet in line with the legs.
2. Exhaling, push back with your hands while raising your hips. Press your heels down towards the ground, keeping your knees slightly bent. Distribute your weight evenly between hands and feet, so that your body forms an inverted 'V'. Push your chest forward through your arms so that your back can arch, with chest aiming towards legs. Relax your head and neck, or bring your chin toward your chest with eyes looking

towards navel. Keep lower abdomen pressed in towards spine. Inhaling, return to all fours.

Repeat this dynamic motion three or four times, aiming to straighten your legs a little more each time. If you are comfortable with the dynamic version, move on to the static version, holding the Dog Stretch.

Static version: ☀ ☀
the Downward-facing Dog Stretch

3. Hold the Dog Stretch, aiming to straighten your legs with heels pressed towards or into the ground.

Timing: Hold for three to eight breaths. Focus your attention on keeping your hips lifted and your weight evenly distributed between your hands and feet. To recover, reverse the path taken into the posture and rest for a few recovery breaths in the Child's pose (p149). It is helpful to repeat this exercise two or three times, alternating legs and moving into the extended version on the second or third repetition.

Preparation: Urdhva Mukha Svanasana (Upward-facing Dog Stretch) ☀ ☀ ☀

Prepare by executing the Cobra (Bhujangasana, p86)

1. Lie flat on your abdomen, placing hands alongside your chest with elbows bent and at your sides. Rest your chin on the ground. Legs are straight and together or a small distance apart and toes point out behind you.
2. Inhaling, press palms and tops of your feet into the ground as you raise your chest, hips and knees and straighten your arms. Reach your chin and head, stretching the front of your neck and torso as you bend backwards. Keep your shoulders down, so that your neck is long and your chest

open. Keep your legs parallel, so your weight rests on the centre of the tops of the feet, with your toes pointing behind you. Hold for three to eight breaths. To recover, lower your knees, then torso, as you return to your abdomen.

Options for holding Urdhva Mukha Svanasana

A. Place your hands on blocks to raise your body higher off the ground. The benefits of this posture are the same as for the Cobra.
B. Curl your toes under instead of pointing them out, so that you balance on the balls of your feet.

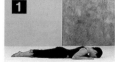 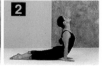 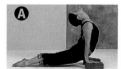 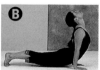

Cautions

- If you have high blood pressure or a heart condition, do the Downward-facing Dog Stretch against a wall, so that your head remains above the level of your heart. This version is also good as preparation and is useful during pregnancy.

- Before you attempt the Upward-facing Dog Stretch (see above), you must be able to do the Cobra.
- If you have a back problem, warm up your spine well by doing the Cat Stretch (p83). When you execute the Dog Stretch, do so with caution.

URDHVA DHANURASANA
The Full Bridge
अर्ध्व धनुरासन

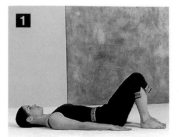

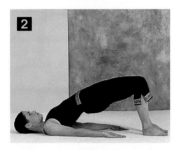

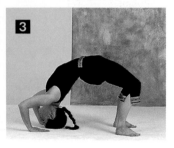

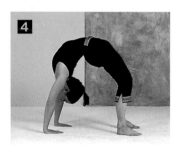

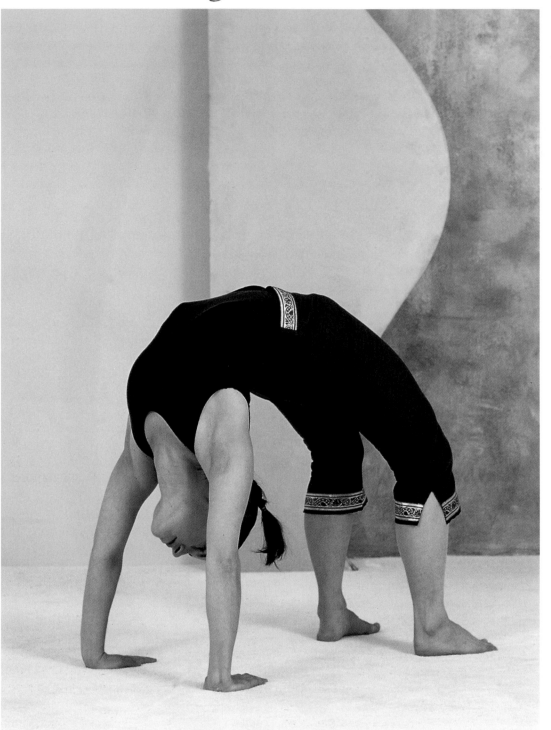

Benefits

- Strengthens the thigh and the buttock muscles.
- Stretches and strengthens the abdominal muscles and tones the organs.
- Stretches the front of the hips, increasing flexibility.

- The Little Bridge particularly nourishes the thyroid gland with a fresh and increased blood supply.
- Helps regulate the metabolism and keep obesity in check.
- Keeps the spine elastic.
- Nourishes the brain with a fresh blood supply.

'Urdhva' means 'upward facing' and 'Dhanurasana' is the Bow – so Urdhva Dhanurasana is an inverted version of Dhanurasana (the Upward-facing Bow). This posture is also referred to as Chakrasana, the Wheel.

Preparation: dynamic version in Setu Bandha Sarvangasana (the Little Bridge) ☀

1. Start lying on your back, with your knees bent and the soles of your feet on the ground, a small distance apart. Bring your heels in as close as you can to your buttocks. Place your hands on the ground, palms down, with your arms straight and held in at your sides. Check that your back and head are in a straight line.

2. Inhaling, press down on your feet and press your navel towards the ground as you tilt your pelvis and raise your hips upwards. This involves peeling your spine off the ground vertebra for vertebra, until the weight of your body is shared between your feet and shoulders with your chest raised towards your chin. Keep your legs parallel.

   Exhaling, return to the starting position, reversing the motion, by replacing vertebra for vertebra onto the ground as you return to the starting position.

Repeat three to six times dynamically then hold after the inhalation for three to six breaths. Only move on to the Full Bridge if you can comfortably hold the Little Bridge.

The Full Bridge ☀ ☀ ☀

1–2. Start as for Setu Bandha Sarvangasana.

3. Place your hands next to your ears, under your shoulders, with elbows pointing upward and fingers pointing toward your shoulders. Keep your knees bent and your legs parallel. Press down on your hands and place the crown of your head on the ground between your hands.

4. Press down on your hands again and straighten your elbows as you raise your head and shoulders off the ground. Push your chest up and out, to increase the bend in your upper back. Relax your head and neck, with your eyes looking towards the ground.

Timing: Hold for three to eight breaths, focusing on the opening and stretching of your abdomen, chest and throat area. Recover on an exhalation, reversing the path taken on the way into the posture.

Setu Bandha Sarvangasana ☀ ☀ (static version)

1. Start as for the version above, with your arms resting on the ground.

2. Walk your feet in towards your shoulders so that you can take hold of your ankles. Hold as for the static version.

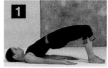 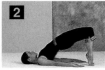 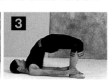

The Half Bridge: dynamic and static versions ☀ ☀

1. Start sitting upright with knees bent and soles on the ground. Hands are at your sides on the ground with fingers facing forward.

2–3. Inhaling, rock your weight forward onto your feet, keeping your legs parallel. Raise your hips as you straighten your elbows, keeping your shoulders pressed down. Head and neck relax downward.

Supported Little Bridge ☀ ☀

A. Place your hands under your lower back and hold as for Setu Bandha Sarvangasana. Fingers support your lower back and thumbs are placed at the sides of your waist.

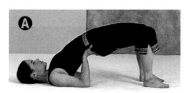

Exhaling, reverse the path to the sitting position.
Repeat three to eight times, then hold in the static version after the inhalation for three to eight breaths.

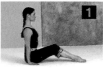 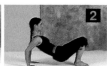 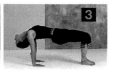

Cautions

- If you have a neck injury or problem, do only the Little Bridge, as the neck rests on the ground. Only do the Half Bridge if you keep your head and neck in line with the rest of your spine, so that your eyes look upwards.
- Keep your legs and feet parallel.

- Move smoothly and slowly into and out of these positions. Never jerk the spine.
- Keep your shoulders pressed down, away from your ears, so that your neck feels long.
- The Full Bridge is an inverted posture and should not be done if you have high blood pressure or a heart condition.

Summary: spinal twists

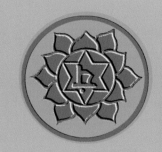

Jathara Parivartanasana, p100

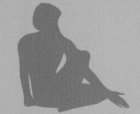

Ardha Matsyendrasana, p102

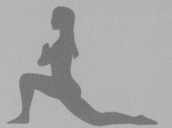

Chandrasana, p104

SITTING POSTURES
Spinal twists

Spinal twists are particularly effective for aligning the spinal vertebrae, twisting the spinal column all the way down to the lumbar region. They give a gentle massage to the internal organs of the abdominal area, allowing a fresh blood supply to nourish the area. They also open the chest area, encouraging fuller breathing, particularly into the ribcage.

The autonomous nervous system

Spinal twists revitalize the nerve ganglia of the autonomic nervous system, which run from the spine to the periphery of the body. They exert a greater influence than any other group of postures on the autonomic nervous system, particularly on the Vagus nerve. This has a calming, soothing effect on the body and mind; it is energizing on a physical as well subtle energetic level.

The autonomic nervous system is controlled in the brain stem and the hypothalamus and is responsible for all functions that are carried out largely without our conscious control. Such functions include digestion, respiration, glandular hormonal secretions, the heartbeat and blood circulation and the functions of the kidneys and the liver.

The Vagus nerve

The Vagus nerve is an important part of our body's parasympathetic nervous system, which also affects the sympathetic nervous system.

The parasympathetic nervous system is the calming, relaxing portion of the autonomic nervous system, which serves to balance out the activating, stimulating effect of the sympathetic portion of the nervous system.

The Vagus nerve runs from the brain down the spinal column and ends at the solar plexus; this nerve has been related to the seven energy centres (chakras) through their relationship with the various sympathetic nerve plexuses in the body.

The energy or power generated through the vitalizing of the nerve centre releases energy that may get locked in the body – in this way the energy can be put to better use. This release can be achieved by doing spinal twists that energize the physical and subtle body (related to the chakras).

This interaction is only one example of how work on a physical level can influence other more subtle levels of energy and consciousness.

The nerve plexuses associated with the seven energy centres/chakras are:

- 1st energy centre = Muladhara chakra:
  Sacro-Coccygeal Plexus
- 2nd energy centre = Svadhisthana chakra:
  Prostatic Plexus in men and related to the ovaries
  in women.
- 3rd energy centre = Manipura chakra: Solar Plexus
- 4th energy centre = Anahata chakra: Cardiac/
  Heart Plexus
- 5th energy centre = Visuddha chakra: Laryngeal,
  Pharyngeal Plexus
- 6th energy centre = Ajna chakra: Cavernous Plexus
  (behind and in the space between the brow)
- 7th energy centre = Sahasrara chakra: Pineal gland

Spinal twists benefit all the energy centres, particularly opening the heart centre (Anahata chakra).

JATHARA PARIVARTANASANA
Spinal Twists
जठर परिवर्तनासन

'Jathara' translates as 'abdomen', 'Parivritti' means 'turning around', so Jathara Parivartanasana is a posture that 'turns around' the abdominal area and gives a twist to the spine. There are several versions of these Spinal Twists, each with a different leg, arm or torso position.

Timing: Repeat two to six times, co-ordinating breath with movement. Feel the movement as a relaxed rolling from one side to the other, which gives a gentle massage to the lower back. You can include a head movement on each exhalation, turning your head in the opposite direction to your knee. Use the dynamic versions as preparation for the static version.

After any of these versions, hug both knees into the chest, as in Apanasana (p149) and hold for two to four breaths, to return symmetry to the body after twisting to both sides. You can also hug the knees before you repeat the posture on the other side, particularly if you have a back problem. Move slowly and smoothly into and out of twists, as any sudden jerks can be dangerous for the spine.

Dynamic version

1. Lie on your back with your arms outstretched on the ground at shoulder height, with palms up or down. Bend your knees, placing your soles on the ground as close to your hips as possible. Your legs and feet should be hip distance or more apart. Press your navel down towards the ground, so that your entire spine, including your lower back, is resting on the ground. Check that your spine and head are in a straight line. Inhale and simply feel the length of your spine.
2. Exhaling, lower your knees to the right, keeping both feet and shoulders in contact with the ground. Keep your hips in line with your shoulders – do not allow the twisting action to shift your hips to the side, as the twist must remain around the central axis of your spine. Inhaling, return your knees to the centred starting position. Repeat, lowering your knees to the left.

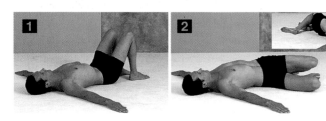

Static version

Hold the twist after each exhalation for two to four breaths. Then, inhaling, to return to the centred starting position.
As you hold the twist, focus your attention on breathing into the open side of your chest.

Option 1: dynamic or static version

1. Start as for the dynamic version, placing both your legs and feet together.
2. When twisting, allow your left foot to come off the ground as you twist to the right, and vice versa. This gives a little more of a twisting action to the spine.

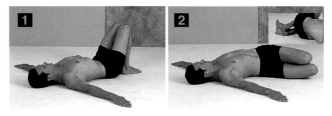

Option 2: dynamic or static version

1. Start as for the previous instructions, placing your legs and feet together and bringing your knees in over your abdomen.
2. When twisting, lower your knees to either side, keeping your legs held together.

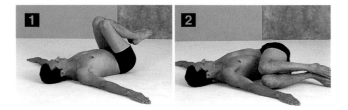

Benefits
- Helps relieve backache.
- Gives a gentle massage to the lower back.
- Aligns the spinal vertebrae.
- Increases a sense of vitality.

- Gives a gentle squeeze to the abdominal organs, such as the stomach, liver, kidneys and pancreas, and helps peristalsis in the intestines.
- Gives a gentle squeeze to the Vagus nerve and the root of the autonomic nervous system.

Option 4: dynamic or static version ☀ ☀ ☀

1. Start as for the previous instructions, with legs and feet together and parallel. Extend your legs to a vertical position, flexing your feet.
2. When twisting, keep your legs together as you lower them. On inhalation, press your arms and hands into the ground to assist your recovery to the starting position. This requires strong abdominal and back muscles.

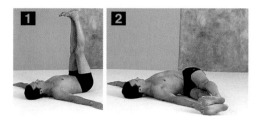

One-legged static version ☀ ☀

1. Start as for the previous instructions, with your right leg straight and left knee bent in over your abdomen.
2. Place your right hand on the outside of your left knee (opposite hand to knee). Your left arm is extended out to the side at shoulder height.

   Exhaling, twist towards the right by lowering your knee to the left. Turn your head to the left. Keep your right leg extended. Keep both shoulders on the ground.

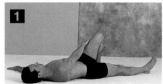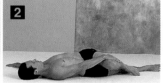

Timing: Hold for two to six breaths, breathing into the open side of your chest. Recover to the starting position on an inhalation and rest for a moment, hugging both knees into your chest with your arms. Repeat the twist to the right, with your right leg bent and your head turned to the right.

Static version lying face-down ☀ ☀ ☀

1. Lie with your forehead on the ground and your legs apart in an inverted 'V'. Flex your feet and curl your toes under. Your left arm extends, palm down, on the ground in front of you. Your right arm extends to the side at shoulder height, palm down. Inhaling, reach forward with your left arm and extend your spine.
2. Exhaling, raise your right arm, shoulder and hip, tracing a semi-circle with your right arm in line with your shoulders.
3. Complete the circle until you can place your right hand on the ground, so that your chest is open facing upward. Eyes and head look over your right shoulder.

   Keep your left arm where it is and both feet on the ground as you twist.

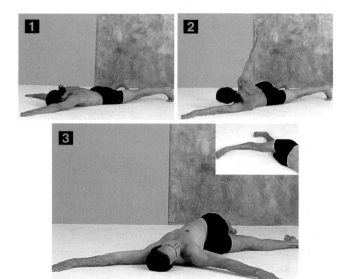

Timing: Hold for three to six breaths, then reverse the path taken into the twist on an inhalation, returning to the starting position. Rest for two or three breaths, then repeat the twist raising your left arm, with your right arm stretched out on the ground in front of you.

Cautions

- Take care if you have a spinal injury or problem. Consult your doctor before doing spinal twists.
- Take care not to jerk into or out of the twist and never bounce while holding a twist.

ARDHA MATSYENDRASANA
Half Twist in a sitting position
अर्ध मत्स्येन्द्रासन

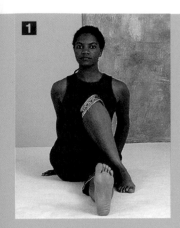

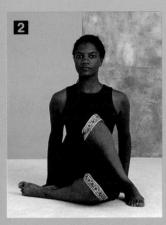

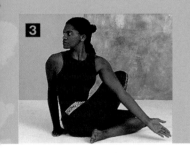

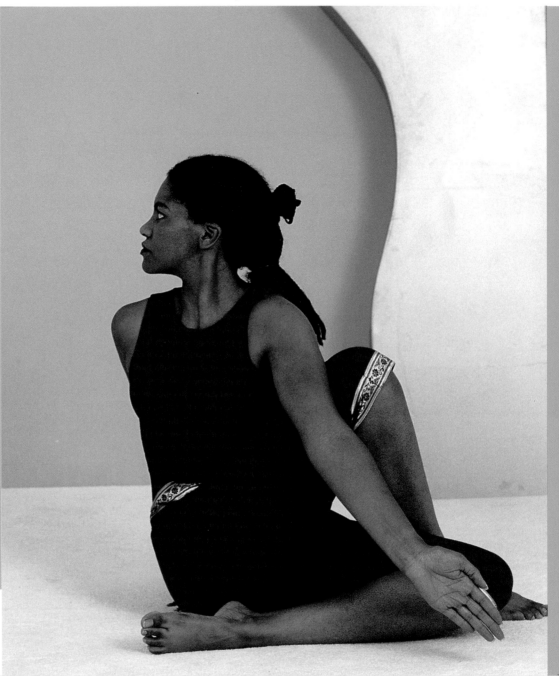

Benefits

- Helps relieve backache and aligns the vertebrae.
- Gives a gentle squeeze to the abdominal organs, such as the stomach, liver, kidneys and pancreas, and helps peristalsis in the intestines.
- Gives a gentle squeeze to the Vagus nerve and the root of the autonomic nervous system.
- Increases sense of vitality.
- Strengthens the back.

Cautions

- Take care if you have a spinal injury or problem, perhaps staying with simpler twist versions. Consult your doctor or physiotherapist before doing spinal twists.
- Do no jerk into or out of the twist and never force a twist.
- Keep your spine lengthened and centred throughout, so that your spine forms a central axis for your twist.
- Remain sitting with weight on both buttocks throughout.
- Keep your shoulders level throughout.

'Ardha' means 'half' and 'Matsyendrasana' is the name of a great Yogi. It also translates as the 'lord of fish', as this twisting posture is said to have first been taught by a fish who wished to be transformed into a human by Lord Shiva. 'Matsya' also translates as 'the power that vitalizes and energizes and has the ability to turn on the subtle energies of the body and mind'. 'Endra' refers to the power of the mind. Thus this posture is one of the most powerful exercises to increase mental alertness and clarity.

Ardha Matsyendrasana ☀☀

1. Sit with your back upright, your left leg extended and your right leg bent. Place the sole of your right foot on the ground outside your left leg. Press your right shin against your left knee or thigh. Bring your right heel in as close as possible to your left hip.
2. Bend your left leg so that your outer thigh rests on the ground; your left heel is close to your buttocks.

3. Inhaling, extend up through your spine and head as you place your right hand at the base of your spine, on the ground behind you.
   Place your left arm on the outer side of your right thigh, holding your left arm straight out and with your palm facing forward.
   Turn your head and eyes to look over your right shoulder. Keep your shoulders level throughout.

Timing: Hold for three to eight breaths, keeping your spine centred and lengthened. Breathe into the open side (the right side, in this case) of your chest. To recover, exhale, reversing your path. Repeat to the other side. After twisting both ways, rest for two to five breaths in a symmetrical counter-posture, such as Apanasana (p149) or Pascimottanasana (p72).

Preparation: sitting on a chair ☀

A. Sit sideways on a chair with a backrest, so that the backrest is on your right. Place your feet flat on the ground (or on a pile of books if your feet do not reach the ground). Gently turn your torso to the right, taking hold of the backrest. Turn your head and eyes to look over your right shoulder.
    Hold for three to six breaths. Then sit on the other side of the chair and repeat the twist to the left.

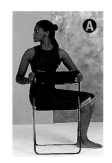

Extra preparation ☀☀

1–3. Execute as for Ardha Matsyendrasana, but allow your left leg to remain extended with your foot flexed.

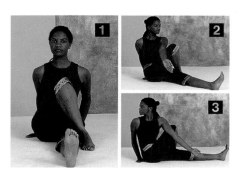

Half Lotus Half Twist ☀☀☀

1. Begin as for Ardha Matsyendrasana, with your left leg straight and the foot flexed. Place your right leg into Padmasana (the Half Lotus), with your right heel in your left groin.
2. While inhaling, lengthen your spine, pulling back in your right shoulder and arm and wrapping your right arm around the back of your waist, so that you can hold your right foot in your right hand.
3–4. Place your left hand on the outside of your right thigh, so that your torso is twisted, straightening your left arm, with palm either facing forward or placed on your right thigh. Turn to look over your right shoulder. Hold as for Ardha Matsyendrasana.
    Repeat to the other side, then move into a symmetrical counter-posture.

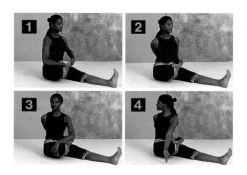

CHANDRASANA
The Crescent Moon
चन्द्रासन

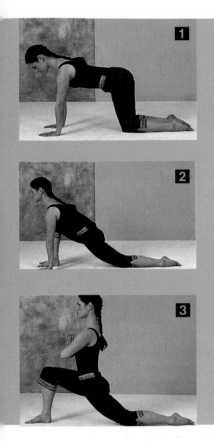

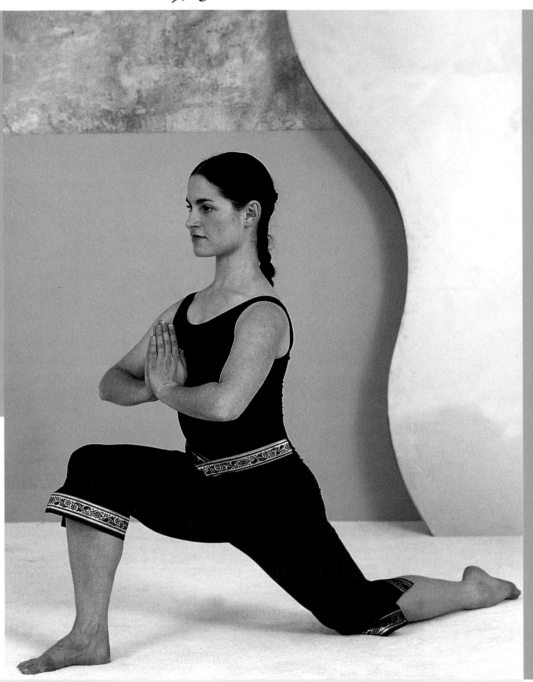

Benefits

- Stretches, limbers and tones the legs and hips.
- Relaxes the adductor (inner thigh) muscles.
- Increases the blood supply to the pelvic area.
- Gives a gentle squeeze to the colon on the side where the leg is forward. This helps peristalsis and elimination.
- Can prevent and relieve sciatica.

Cautions

- Do not bounce while holding or moving into the Crescent Moon.
- Do not over-stretch in this posture, as you may pull or strain a muscle.
- Try to keep your spine extended and your hips as square as possible throughout.

The Crescent Moon and the Pigeon are used as preparatory exercises for Hanumanasana (the Splits). These postures are not always considered to be spinal twists, but they do involve a twist in the lumbar spine in order to hold the back leg behind the body, while aiming to keep the hips as square as possible.

The Crescent Moon ☀

1. Kneel on all fours, with toes pointing out behind you.
2. Bring your right leg forward, placing your foot flat on the ground, with toes pointing forward. Your right heel is placed directly under your right knee, so that your right leg forms a right angle. Lunge forward into your left hip, feeling a stretch across the front of your left hip.

Your hands and fingers are placed on either side of your right foot, with fingers pointing forward.

3. If you feel your balance is stable, bring your torso into an upright position and place your hands in the Prayer pose. Press down your shoulders as you reach forward with your head, so that your spine is stretched out. Your eyes look forward, in front of you.

Timing: Hold this position for four to eight breaths.
To recover, reverse the path taken into the position. Repeat with the left leg forward. After stretching both sides, rest in the Child's pose (p149) for a few recovery breaths, to rest and to restore symmetry to the body.

Crescent Moon in a backward bend ☀☀☀

Start in the Crescent Moon (step 3), with your hands in the Prayer pose.

A. Inhaling, stretch your arms up next to your ears, parting your hands and reaching them backwards. Allow your spine to bend backwards, taking your head with you and looking back toward your hands.

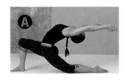

The Splits (Hanumanasana) ☀☀☀

Start as for the Crescent Moon, keeping your hands on the ground on either side of your front foot.

1. Slide your back leg away from your torso, aiming to straighten both legs. Using your hands on the ground for support, lower your hips as close as you can to the ground.
   Hold for four to eight breaths.

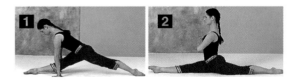

2. If you are in the Full Splits, bring your hands into the Prayer pose at your sternum. Repeat with your other leg forward. After doing both sides, move into a symmetrical counter-posture such as Upavista Konasana (p74) or the Child's pose (p149) for three to eight breaths.

The Pigeon (Eka Pada Rajakapotasana) ☀☀

1. Start kneeling, then extend your left leg behind you, keeping it in line with your left hip. Your left knee faces down, with the foot extended. Sit to the outside of your right foot and leg, so that your right heel is close in to the left side of your groin. Place your fingertips on the ground in front of you, with arms straight and back upright and your hips and shoulders facing as squarely as possible to the front.

   Hold this position for four to eight breaths. After repeating to the other side, move into a symmetrical counter-posture, such as the Child's pose.

2. If you are able to comfortably hold this position, sit with your back to a wall, so that when you bend your left leg up from the knee, your left knee and foot rest against the wall.

3. Bend backwards, bringing your head towards your left foot. If you can comfortably achieve this, take hold of your left foot with both hands, with elbows raised and arms reaching overhead. Use your hands to ease your foot closer in towards your head. If you can comfortably hold this position against a wall, move on to attempt it away from a wall.

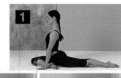
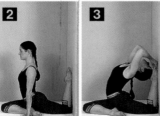

Summary: standing postures

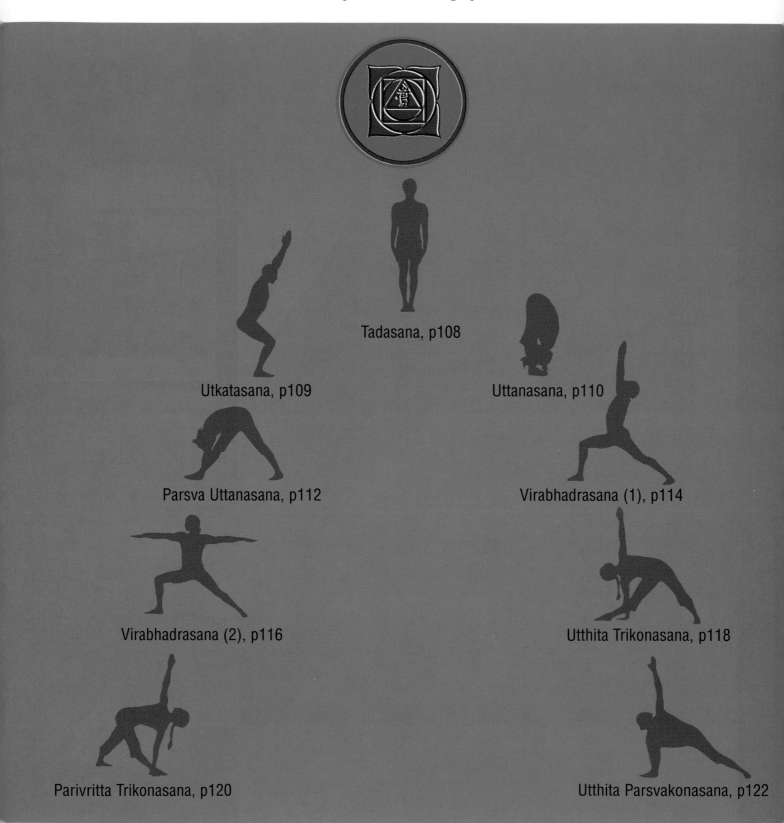

Tadasana, p108

Utkatasana, p109

Uttanasana, p110

Parsva Uttanasana, p112

Virabhadrasana (1), p114

Virabhadrasana (2), p116

Utthita Trikonasana, p118

Parivritta Trikonasana, p120

Utthita Parsvakonasana, p122

Counter-postures are essential to all postures in

Yoga, including the asymmetrical standing postures. The aim of a counter-pose is to restore symmetry in the body after executing these asymmetrical standing postures, and they also give your legs and spine a relaxing stretch.

Counter-postures for asymmetrical standing postures

After doing both sides of an asymmetrical standing posture, return your feet and body to a centred position, facing the front. Spread your legs apart and bring your feet into a parallel position. Keep your knees straight or slightly bent.

1. Bend forward from your hips, allowing your arms to hang down. If you have high blood pressure or a heart condition, bend halfway forward, placing your hands against a wall for support, so your head is in line with your spine.

Options for arms

2. Fold your arms in front of your body while you are upright. As you bend forward, allow your folded arms to hang down toward the ground.

3. Place your hands flat on the ground in the forward bend.

Timing: Hold for three or four recovery breaths, or for a third of the time that you held the asymmetrical posture.

Other counter-posture options

- Hold Tadasana or Samasthiti.
- Move into a rest pose such as Savasana or the Child's pose.

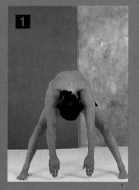

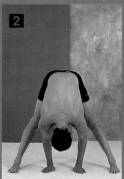

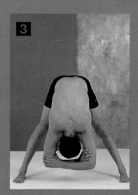

TADASANA
The Mountain

ताड़ासन

Tadasana is a development on Samasthiti – it is also known as Stambhasana, the Pillar.
This posture cultivates a sense of strength and stability. Because the quality of stability is an important part of any foundation, Tadasana is used as a starting position for almost all standing postures. It also is advised as a posture in its own right, as part of your Yoga session. Tadasana can be included at various stages in a session and as a symmetrical counter-posture to standing postures.

Timing: Hold for four to eight breaths.

Samasthiti (the most basic standing position)

Literally, 'sama' translates as 'upright' or 'erect', and 'sthiti' translates as 'steady' or 'in steadiness'. Samasthiti thus refers to a relaxed and steady standing position.

The aim of this posture, as a starting position, is to achieve attention without tension that will be carried over to the postures that follow. Samasthiti is alive and poised, rather than rigid or tense – this is achieved by feeling that you are growing ever taller, floating upwards through the crown of your head, while feeling grounded through your feet and legs.

Samasthiti allows you to find balance in your body, with your weight evenly distributed on both sides, before moving into a posture. From a good starting position, the standing postures and balances will be easier to execute and you will be less likely to injure yourself. Flow of movement and breathing will also be greatly assisted.

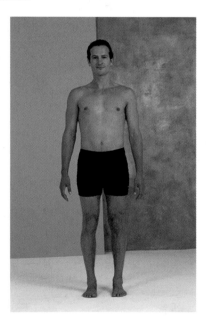

Tadasana – the Mountain

This posture is effective in bringing your awareness to how your mind and imagination influence and literally sway your posture and balance.

You will notice a natural tendency to sway while holding any standing position. The idea is to gently control this natural sway in order to improve your balance, mental focus and willpower. One way to do this is to focus your attention on a sense of gently growing taller. Focusing your eyes can also help – you will notice it is more difficult (although good practice) to find your balance with your eyes closed. A stable starting position will help you to keep your balance steady in the postures that follow – and don't forget to breathe.

- Stand with your feet and legs together.
- Knees are pulled up into your thighs and heels and big toe joints are touching.
- Squeeze your legs together to form a strong, supportive pillar for the rest of your body.
- Further lengthen your spinal column and the back of your neck, keeping your chin parallel to the ground.
- Press your abdomen into your spine.
- Breathe into your chest area, expanding the front and back of your ribcage on inhalation.
- Pull down in your shoulders, reaching downward through your arms, hands and fingers. Take care to keep your chest open and arms held at your sides.
- The idea is that there is a feeling of lengthening up through the central column of your body and reaching down through your arms.

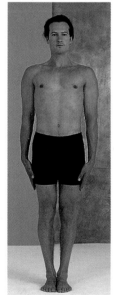

UTKATASANA
The Squat

उत्कटासन

The word 'utkata' means 'powerful', 'fierce', 'mighty' or 'uneven'. Utkatasana is a posture that forms a zig zag shape with the body, with heels, hips and arms extending in opposite directions as if aiming to sit on an imaginary chair. This posture builds power and strength in the body.

Dynamic Squat ☀

1. Start in Tadasana.
2. Inhaling, stretch your arms overhead, so that they are parallel with your hands; fingers pointing upward. You could also hold your arms in the Prayer pose overhead, with thumbs interlinked; or with your arms extended and reaching forward in front of you, at shoulder height, with hands clasped (A).
3. Exhaling, bend your knees as much as you can, keeping your heels pressed into the ground and your legs and knees together. Keep your spine, chest, head and arms lifted and extending diagonally upwards. Your torso will naturally bend forward slightly. Hold your abdomen in toward your spine. Inhaling, straighten your legs and return to the upright position
Repeat four to eight times.

Static Squat ☀

Move into the static version, as for the dynamic version, holding after the exhalation, for four to eight breaths. After inhaling to return to the upright position, exhale, lowering your arms back to your sides, returning to the starting position in Tadasana. Repeat two or three times if you wish, then relax in Samasthiti (p108) for a few recovery breaths.

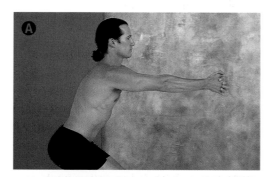

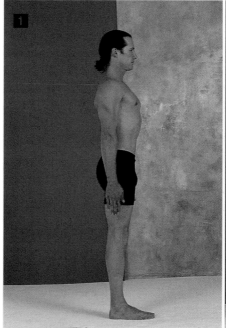

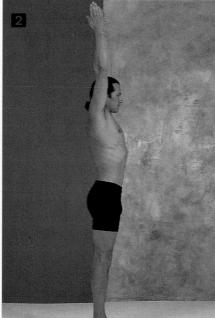

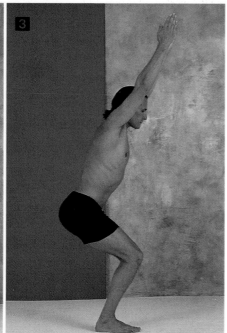

Benefits

- Stretches the Achilles tendon and strengthens the thigh muscles.
- Strengthens and increases mobility in the ankle, knee and hip joints.
- Loosens the shoulder joints.
- Tones and strengthens the back muscles.
- Promotes better body alignment and the even muscular development on both sides of the body.

- Gently massages the lungs and heart by the movement of the diaphragm.
- Assists digestion and elimination.
- Good to do during pregnancy.

Cautions

- If you are pregnant, stand with your legs slightly apart, taking care to keep your legs parallel throughout.
- Do not hold your breath while holding the posture.

UTTANASANA
Standing Forward Bend
उत्तानासन

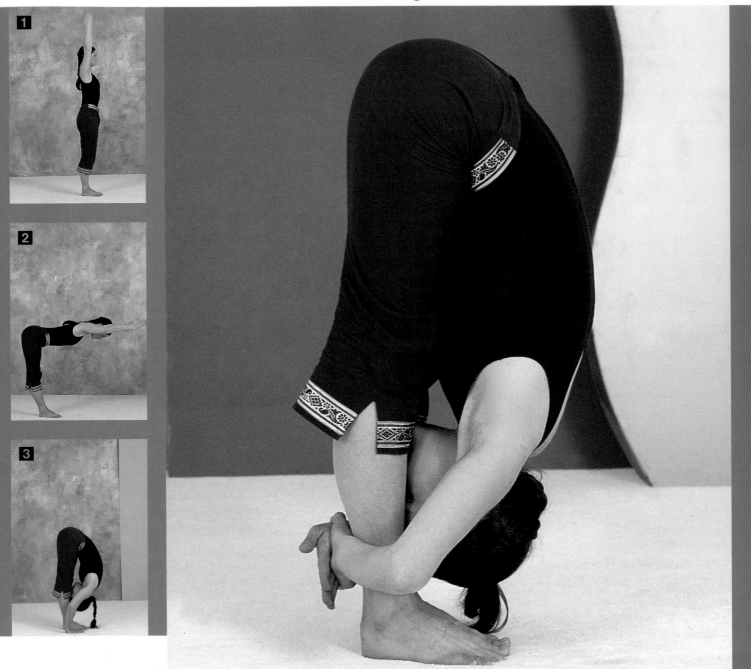

Benefits

- Has all the benefits of Pascimottanasana (p72)
- Particularly benefits the sacral area of the spine, although it gives a stretch to the entire spinal column.
- Strengthens and stretches the hamstrings.
- Gives a gentle massage to the abdominal organs, such as the liver and spleen, and aids digestion.
- Tones the kidneys.
- Tones the nervous system.

- Helpful in depression, to freshen the mind and enhance energy levels.
- Generally has an energizing and refreshing effect on the mind and body.
- Increases blood supply to the head area and brain, helping to prevent wrinkles by bringing a fresh blood supply to the facial tissues.
- Offers all the benefits of inverted postures.
- Cultivates a state of peace in the mind.

'Tan' means 'to stretch' or 'lengthen out' and 'ut' refers to an attitude of being deliberate or intense. This posture offers a deliberate and intense stretch to the spine and the back of the legs. Uttanasana has different names, depending on the position of the hands: Padangusthasana refers to holding the big toe; Padahastasana refers to the placing of the hands under the balls of the feet. In Uttanasana, the hands are placed alongside the feet. Standing postures are more strenuous than sitting postures, so prepare as for Parsva Uttanasana (p112) with a Sitting Forward Bend, such as Pascimottanasana.

Dynamic version ☀☀

1. Start in Tadasana, with feet together or hip distance apart. Squeeze your legs together in the parallel position throughout. Inhaling, stretch your arms overhead, placing your arms next to your ears, with your fingers pointing upwards and palms facing each other.
2. Exhaling, reach forwards and then down with your torso, keeping your arms next to your ears, to assist you to keep your spine extended with your head and neck in line with your spine.
3. When you can bend no further without rounding your spine, place your hands around the outsides of your ankles or flat on the ground alongside your feet – whatever level you are able to reach comfortably. The legs are straight or slightly bent.

Use your arms to help ease chest and head toward your legs, keeping your torso centred between your legs. Inhaling, reverse the path until you are upright, initiating the movement by extending your spine and stretching your arms forward as you replace them next to your ears. Repeat the dynamic motion three to eight times. This can be used in preparation for the static version.

Static version ☀☀☀

4. Execute as for the dynamic version, aiming to keep your legs as straight as possible. If you wish to extend the position, place your hands behind your ankles and take hold of your left wrist in your right hand. The weight of your body is over the balls of your feet.

Timing: For the static version, hold after the first exhalation for three to eight breaths. Breathe into your ribcage, particularly focusing on breathing into the back of your ribcage and chest. Recover as for the dynamic version, on an inhalation, making sure to bring your arms next to your ears to initiate the recovery so that your spine is straightened out.

Options for hands

- Hold your ankles or place your hand behind your knees.

Dynamic or static versions in ☀☀☀ Padangusthasana or Padahastasana

Start as for Uttanasana.

A. For Padangusthasana, take hold of your big toes in the forward bend, opening out your elbows to assist you.
B. For Padahastasana, place your palms underneath the balls of your feet, opening your elbows out to the sides.
C. For the dynamic version of either posture, on inhalation and

without adjusting your hands, extend your spine, straighten your arms and raise your chin and head to look out in front of you. On exhalation, return to the Full Forward Bend.

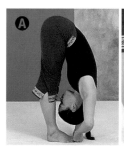
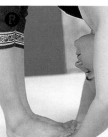
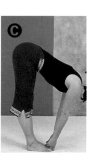

Cautions

- If you suffer from any condition where your head should not be below the level of your heart, bend only half way, placing your hands against a wall for support.
- If you find you take strain in the Forward Bend with straight legs, practice with legs slightly bent.

- Prepare with Sitting Forward Bends, such as Pascimottanasana (p72), before attempting a Standing Forward Bend.
- Remember to breathe while holding the Forward Bend, focusing on breathing into the back of the ribcage. Recover slowly and with care.

PARSVA UTTANASANA
Sideways-facing Forward Bend
पार्श्व उत्तानासन

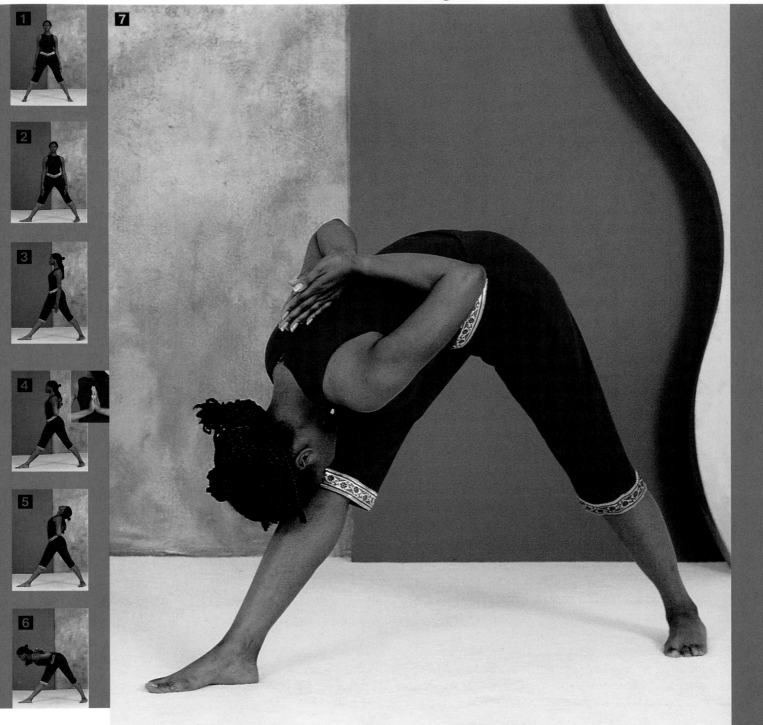

Benefits
- Stretches and strengthens the spine.
- Tones the nervous system.
- Stretches the hamstrings.
- Strengthens and tones the muscles of the legs.
- Increases blood supply to the head and face.
- Gently massages the organs in the abdomen, assisting digestion and elimination.
- Gives a gentle massage to the kidneys.
- Is energizing and refreshing.

"Parsva' means sideways and 'Uttan' means 'extended' or 'stretched'. This posture is a version of Uttanasana that some people find easier, as the legs form a wider and thus more stable base – it may also be called Parsvottanasana.

Moving into Parsva Uttanasana

1. Start in Tadasana and spread your legs apart, keeping your feet parallel and both heels in line with each other.
2. Turn your right foot out to the side at a 90° angle and your left foot also to the right, at a 45° angle.
3. Turn your entire body to face the right side, without adjusting the position of your feet. Keep your shoulders over your hips, so that you face squarely to the side. The weight of your body should be evenly distributed over both legs, with knees locked for stability.
4. Place your hands in the Prayer pose behind your back.
5. Inhaling, stretch up with your chest, neck and chin, extending your upper torso into a slight upper back bend.
6. Exhaling, with spine extended, bend forward from your hips.
7. Keep your spine extended for as long as possible, before rounding it to bring your head down toward your leg.

Timing: Hold for three to six breaths.
To recover, return to the centred starting position, facing the front with your feet parallel. Repeat to the left. After working on both sides, move into a symmetrical counter-posture to restore symmetry to the body.

Options for arms

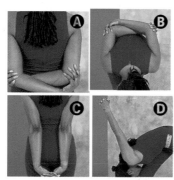

A&B. Fold your arms behind your back, taking hold of your elbows or forearms.

C&D. Clasp your hands behind your back with your arms straight. As you bend forward, raise your arms toward your head.

Dynamic or static version

Position your body, legs and feet for Parsva Uttanasana, starting with your arms at your sides.

1. Inhaling, raise your arms overhead, with arms parallel and placed next to your ears. Palms face each other with fingers pointing upwards.
2. Exhaling, keep your arms next to your ears and your spine extended as you bend forward over your right leg, bringing your torso and head as close to your leg as possible.
3. When you can bend no further without rounding your spine,

place your hands alongside your right foot or take hold of your right ankle. Ease your head toward your leg, using your arms for assistance. Aim to keep your hips square by pulling back and up in your hip. Take care to distribute your weight evenly on both legs, with feet firmly planted onto the ground.

Inhaling, extend your spine, replacing your arms next to your ears, then reverse the path taken into the forward bend to return to an upright position.

Repeat two to four times in a smooth and flowing manner, then repeat to the other side.

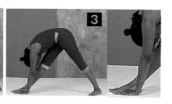

Static version

Execute as for the dynamic version, holding after exhalation for three to six breaths.

Cautions

- The Full Forward Bend is an inverted posture, so if you suffer from a heart condition, high blood pressure or any eye condition where your head should not be held below the level of your heart, only do half the Forward Bend (perhaps resting your hands against a wall for support). If your arms are in the extended position, keep your arms next to your ears, so that your spine, neck and head are in alignment.

- Prepare with sitting forward bends before attempting a standing forward bend.
- If you find you take strain in the forward bend with straight legs, practise a few times with a slightly bent front leg in preparation for the full forward bend.
- Remember to breathe while holding the forward bend and to recover with care.
- Do a symmetrical counter-posture after stretching both sides, in order to restore symmetry to the body.

VIRABHADRASANA (1)
The Warrior
वीरभद्रासन १

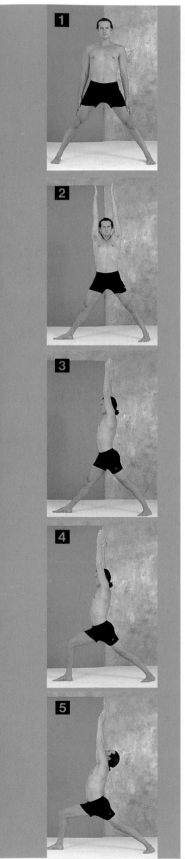

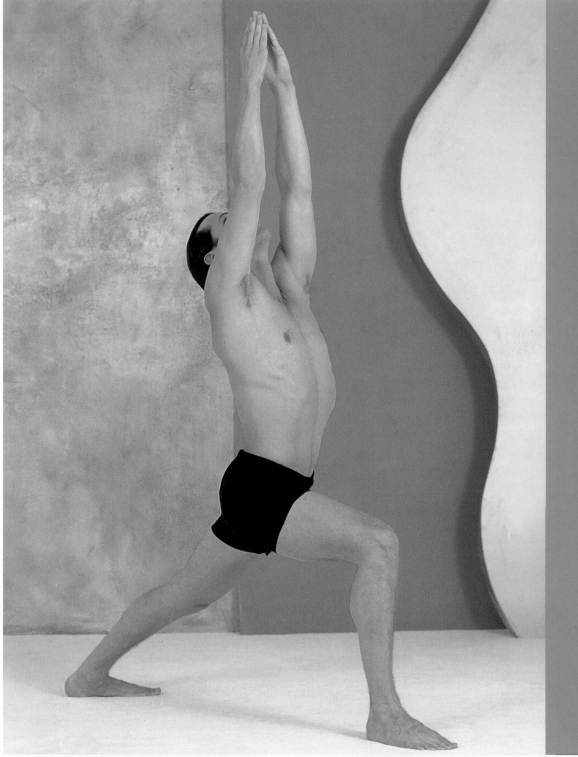

Benefits (Virabhadrasana 1 & 2)

- Strengthens, firms and tones the legs, hips, abdomen, back and neck muscles.
- Enhances the sense of balance on both sides of the body.
- Limbers and strengthens the ankles, knees, hips and shoulders.
- Expands the chest, encouraging deeper breathing.
- Improves balance and concentration.

'Virabhadra' is the name of a powerful hero in a Hindu legend, and this posture is said to cultivate heroic strength in the body and mind. There are three versions of the posture – two are presented on this and the following page, while the third, a balancing posture, is on p128.

Dynamic Virabhadrasana (1) ☀☀

1. Start in Tadasana and spread your legs as far apart as you can, while retaining your stability. Keep your heels in line with each other.
2. Inhaling, raise your arms overhead, stretching your arms, hands and fingers upward and keeping your arms parallel. Keep your shoulders pressed down and your chest open.
3. Breathe naturally as you position your feet and legs. Turn your right leg and foot out to point sideways at a 90° angle to the front. Turn your left foot in at a 45° angle. Keep both legs straight with heels securely planted onto the ground. Turn your hips and body to face squarely to the right, without adjusting the position of your feet. Inhaling, stretch up from your waist through your arms.
4. Exhaling, begin to bend your right knee, aiming to place your thigh parallel to the ground. Take care to keep your right knee facing forward, so that your knee is positioned over your heel and your instep is lifted.
   Keep your abdomen lifted and strive for a feeling of stretching your head, chest and hands upwards. Keep your shoulders over your hips and keep both as square as possible. Your torso should be vertical and centred. Lift out of your hips by lifting your abdominal muscles.
5. Alternate inhalation and straightening your right leg with exhalation and bending your right leg into Virabhadrasana. Take care to keep your spine extended throughout and your abdominal muscles lifted.
   Repeat four to eight times, ending on an inhalation, with legs straightening. Then return to the centred starting position, facing the front.
   Repeat to the left. This serves as a good warm-up for the static version.

Static Virabhadrasana (1) ☀☀

5. Execute the posture as for the dynamic version, but hold after exhaling into the position, looking up toward your hands, with chin reaching upward stretching the front of your neck.
   Keep your spine and the back of your neck extended. Aim to form a right angle with your right leg.

Timing for static version: Hold after exhaling into the position for four to eight breaths. Recover by reversing the path taken into the posture and repeat to the left.

Options for arms

A. Stretch your arms overhead, meeting in the Prayer pose with your thumbs interlocked and fingers touching.
B. Interlock your fingers, stretch and position your palms facing upward.

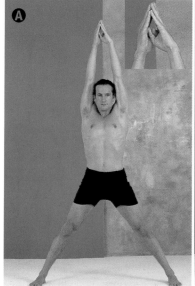
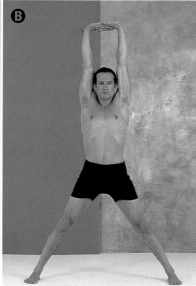

VIRABHADRASANA (2)
The Warrior
वीरभद्रासन २

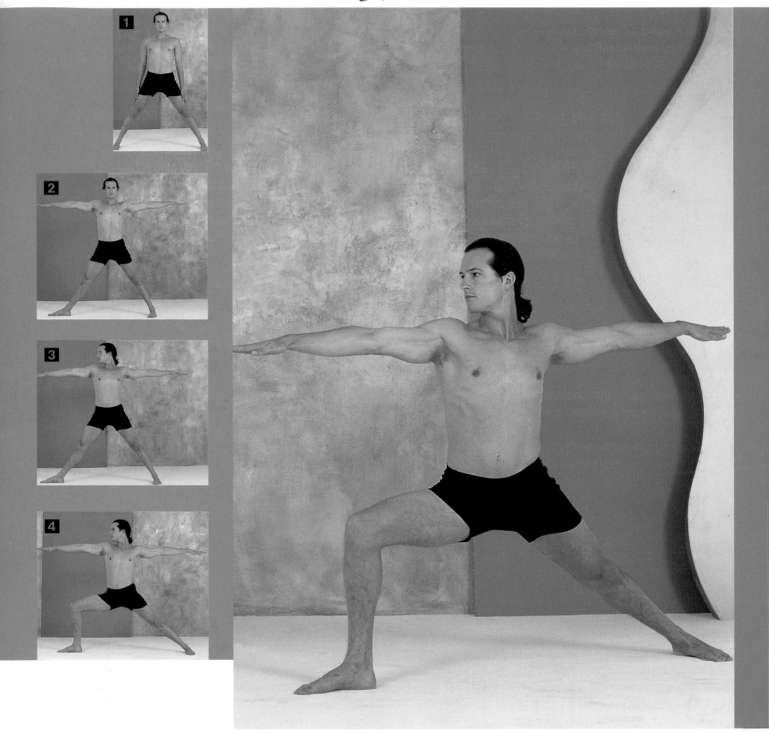

Dynamic Virabhadrasana (2) ☀☀

1. Start facing the front with your legs and feet positioned as for Virabhadrasana 1. Take care to keep both legs straight, with heels pressing into the ground.

2. Raise your arms to your sides at shoulder height, with palms facing down and fingers pointing out to the sides.

3. Inhaling, extend your spine and head upward, growing taller in the posture. Turn your head to the right, to look over your right hand.

4. Exhaling, bend your right knee, taking care to keep your knee pointing out to the side, so that it is positioned over your right heel with the instep of your right foot lifted. Aim to form a right angle with your right leg, with both feet well planted on the ground. Keep your shoulders in line with your hips both squarely facing the front. Pull back in your hip to assist the alignment of your hips to the front. Take care to keep your torso vertical and centred.

   Your arms remain extended in opposite directions, forming one straight and level line from right to left fingertips. Keep your shoulders pressed down, level and relaxed throughout. Inhaling, straighten your right knee and leg, maintaining the alignment of your body, feet and head.

   Exhaling, bend your right knee, returning into the posture. Repeat three to six times, alternating the final two instructions for inhalation and exhalation, bending and straightening your right leg.

   End on an inhalation, straightening your leg, returning your head to the front. Return your feet into the parallel starting position and repeat to the left. The dynamic version serves as a good warm-up in preparation for the static version.

Static Virabhadrasana (2) ☀☀

Execute as for the dynamic version, holding after exhalation into the position.

Timing: For the static version, hold after exhalation into the position for three to eight breaths.
Keep your heels well planted into the ground throughout and both arms reaching out in opposite directions.
To recover, inhale, straightening your right leg and return to the centred position. Repeat to the left, then move into a symmetrical counter-posture.

Cautions (Virabhadrasana 1 & 2)

• This pose can be strenuous, so take care if you have a heart condition, a weak heart or high blood pressure, or if you simply find yourself straining to hold the posture. Either hold for a shorter period of time, like two or three breaths, or stay with the dynamic version, repeating two or three times. It is less strenuous to hold your hands on your hips throughout, with elbows pointing out to the sides, so that the work in the posture is focused on your legs and hips.

• Do not strain while holding Virabhadrasana. Check your face, throat and abdomen for signs of tension. Also check that your breathing is easy and regular. If you do feel strain, gently move into a counter-posture and take a few recovery breaths.

• Take care not to spread your legs too wide apart. You should be able to keep both heels on the ground and feel comfortable in the position.

• Move into a counter-posture after working on both sides to restore symmetry to your body.

UTTHITA TRIKONASANA
The Extended Triangle

अधित त्रिकोणासन

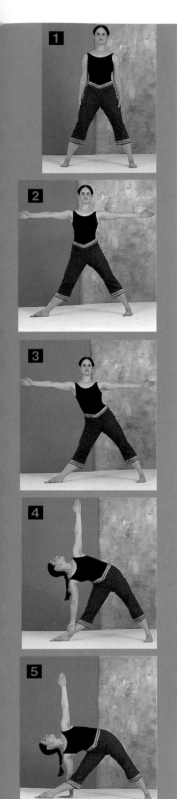

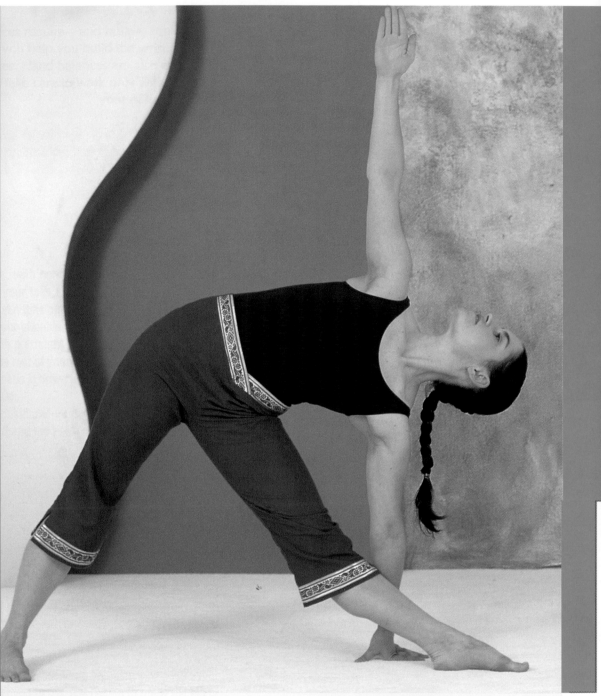

Benefits

- Gives a lateral stretch to the spine.
- Increases hip, shoulder and leg flexibility.
- Helps to firm and tone the leg muscles.
- Helps to remove fat from the waistline.
- When bending to the left, it gives a gentle squeeze to the organs on that side of the abdominal cavity, such as the spleen. When bending to the right, it gives a gentle squeeze to the liver.
- Expands the chest by opening up the ribcage on the side of the raised arm. This posture benefits the Anahata chakra (the heart energy centre).
- Tones the nerves around the spine by stretching out the spine.

The word 'utthita' means 'extended' or 'stretched' and 'trikona' means 'triangle', and this posture creates a few triangles with the body and legs. Trikonasana mainly serves to train awareness of body alignment, as it is one of the few postures that allows the body to bend sideways.

Preparation: using a wall ☀☀

1. Start in Tadasana (p108), with your buttocks and shoulders against a wall. Your feet are parallel and a comfortable distance apart – they should feel well planted flat onto the ground, with even weight distribution between heels and toes.

2. Turn your right foot out at 90° to face the right. Your left foot turns in at 45°, also facing right. Your hips and shoulders face the front and are centred. Lift out of your hips by lifting your abdomen.
   Inhaling, raise both arms to shoulder height, with palms facing forward. Keep your shoulders pressed down and arms and fingers extended, against the wall.

3. Exhaling, reach your arms to the right, keeping them parallel to the ground and shoulders level as you lean. Your hips remain undisturbed. Inhaling, stretch out through your arms and fingers.

4–5. Exhaling, bend sideways, placing your right hand in front of your right leg or on the ground behind your right foot. Do not lean forward or backward or twist your body. Feel your position stabilized by the upward stretch of your left arm with palm facing the front. Your head and eyes look up to your left hand (if you closed your left eye, you should be able to see your left hand out of the right eye).
   If you have a neck problem or find this head position difficult, keep your head facing forward or looking down toward your right foot. Hold while breathing easily. Keep both legs straight with knees locked for stability. To assist in maintaining the alignment of your hips, rotate the tops of your legs forwards.

Utthita Trikonasana without a wall ☀☀☀

Execute as for the version with a wall, except you will not have the wall to help you maintain your stability and alignment.

Timing: Hold for three to eight breaths. Breathe into the open, right side of your chest and focus on keeping your left hip and shoulder opened upwards (or against the wall) and your arms in a straight line.
To recover, on an inhalation reverse the path taken into the position. Then return to the centred standing position and repeat to the left. After stretching both sides, move into a symmetrical counter-posture.

Options for hands

A. Place your hand on a block in front of your right foot.
B. Hold your ankle.
C. Hold the big toe of your right foot between your thumb and the first two fingers of your right hand.
D. Place your hand flat on the ground in front of your right foot.

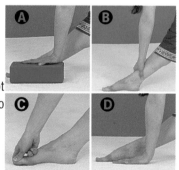

Extended version ☀☀☀

A. To extend the side stretch, reach your left arm overhead to the right side, placing your left arm next to your left ear while keeping arm extended.

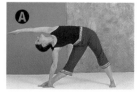

Cautions

• Take care not to bend forward, backward or twist while in the posture.
• Hold your head and neck in line with your spine.
• Try to keep your hips facing to the front throughout, assisted by rotating the tops of the legs forward.
• Bend equally to both sides, to encourage balance on the two sides of the body.

• If you are struggling to balance, practise against the wall to gain confidence in your alignment.
• Prepare for Trikonasana with one of the symmetrical forward bends, then follow Trikonasana with the same forward bend.
• Warm up for side bends with spinal warm-ups and simple side bends.
• Work within your comfortable limits – don't overdo it.

PARIVRITTA TRIKONASANA
The Revolving/Reversed Triangle
परिवृत्त त्रिकोणासन

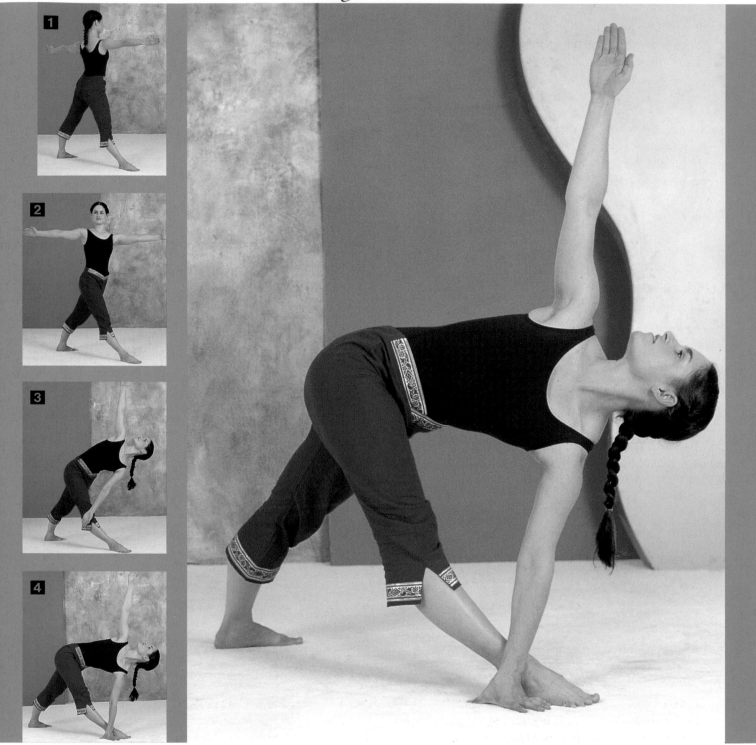

Benefits

- Benefits as for Utthita Trikonasana (p118).
- Tones and strengthens the leg muscles, particularly the thigh, calf and hamstring muscles, as well as the hips.
- Increases the blood supply to the back and spinal nerves through the twisting action.

- Relieves backache and strengthens the back muscles.
- Further expands the chest on the side worked on in Trikonasana when bending to the right.
- Benefits the Anahata chakra (heart centre).
- Gives a gentle squeeze to the abdominal organs and helps to align the spine.

'Parivritta' (also spelled 'parivritta') means 'to reverse' or 'revolve', and 'Trikona' means a triangle. This posture is an extension of Utthita Trikonasana, taking it into a spinal twist. Trikonasana must be well practised before attempting Parivritta Trikonasana. This posture yields greatest benefits when practised directly after Trikonasana and should always be preceded by Trikonasana.

Parivritta Trikonasana ☼ ☼ ☼

1. Start as you would for Trikonasana, with arms raised at your sides at shoulder height. Keep your legs straight and your knees locked for stability. Feet are well planted onto the ground throughout, particularly the heel of your left foot, so that it serves as a stable anchor to help your balance. To feel a greater stability, place your left heel up against a wall.
2. Inhaling, stretch out your spine and lengthen your right leg, pushing down in your right heel as you do so. Revolve your body to the right by rotating your left thigh inward, as you turn to your right.
   Maintain a feeling of lifting out of your hips by lifting your abdomen. Allow your torso, head and arms to follow the revolving action from your hips, twisting around until your chest faces the back wall, with right arm reaching to the left and left arm reaching to the right. Your shoulders remain level, with arms parallel to the ground. Head and eyes face the back. Only twist as far as you feel comfortable.
3. Exhaling, bend from your waist to the left, bringing your left arm down to your right leg, both arms remaining in a straight line.
4. Extend up through the fingers of your right hand. Bend as far as you can, comfortably, placing your left hand on the outside of your right leg or flat on the ground on the inside/ outside of your right foot. Your head and eyes look up to your right hand (which points vertically upwards), so that if you were to close your right eye you would still be able to see your right hand. If your neck is uncomfortable, either look straight out behind you or down toward your left hand. Keep your neck and head in line with the rest of your spine.

Timing: Hold for three to eight breaths, and focus your attention on keeping your spine extended from coccyx through to neck and head. Focus on reaching up through your raised arm; keep your left heel pressing into the ground. Breathe into the side of your chest closest to the ground. To recover, on an inhalation reverse the path taken into the position, in a slow and flowing manner. Move into a counter-posture.

Option for hands

A. Place your hand on a block.

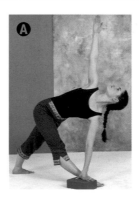

Cautions

- As for Utthita Trikonasana and all spinal twists, take care if you have a back or neck problem
- Take care not to strain in this position – check that your breathing remains easy and that your facial muscles are not tense (smiling helps!).
- Hold your head and neck in line with your spine.
- Do Utthita Trikonasana before Parivritta Trikonasana.
- Always execute a forward-bending counter-posture.
- If you feel any part of your body straining, inhale and slowly recover from the posture, moving into a relaxed counter-posture; take a few recovery breaths.
- Add simple spinal twists to your warm-up of the spine when doing Parivritta Trikonasana.

UTTHITA PARSVAKONASANA
The Extended Sideways Triangle
उत्थित पार्श्वकोणासन

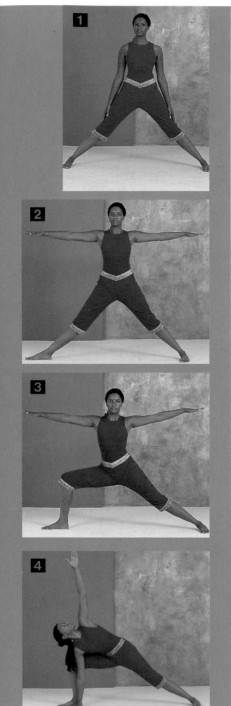

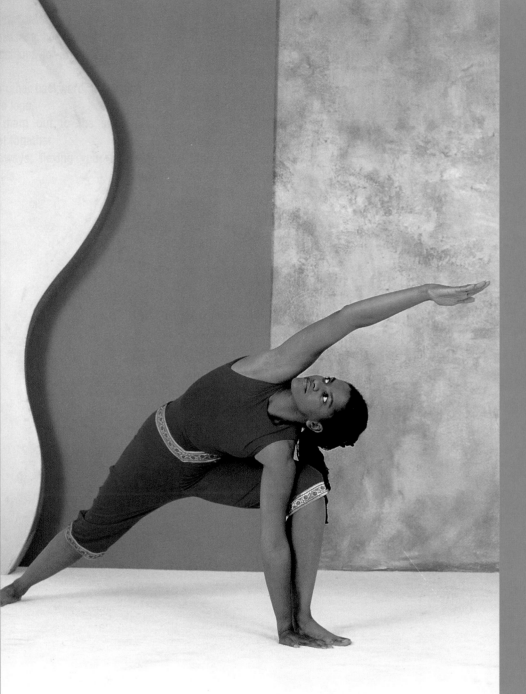

Benefits

- Benefits as for Utthita Trikonasana (p118), with less emphasis on stretching the hamstrings and more emphasis on the lateral bend of the spine and the massage to the abdominal organs.

- Nourishes the spinal column and spinal nerves with a fresh blood supply.
- Expands the chest.
- Increases strength and flexibility in the legs, hips, waist and shoulders.
- Helps tone and trim the waistline.

This is an extended version of Trikonasana, allowing for an extension of the side stretch of the torso. 'Utthita' literally translates as 'extended', 'parsva' mean 'sideways' and 'kona' means 'angle'. The side stretch involves aiming to create a straight line from foot to fingertips, offering a luxurious stretch to each side of the body in turn.

Utthita Parsvakonasana ☀☀

1. Start in Tadasana and spread or jump your legs apart – they should be wider apart than for Trikonasana, but still comfortable.
2. Position your feet by turning your right foot out at 90° (to point to the right) and your left foot in slightly from the parallel position, also pointing to the right. Keep both legs extended. Inhaling, raise your arms sideways to shoulder height, keeping both arms extended.
3. Exhaling, bend your right leg at the knee, aiming to form a right angle (with your right thigh parallel to the ground). Keep your right knee positioned over your right heel (do not allow the knee to fall forward or backward) and keep both feet flat on the ground. Inhaling, feel your stability in the position.
4. Exhaling, bend sideways to the right, placing your right hand on the ground against and in front of your right leg and in line with your right foot. Your left arm points vertically upward, extending through your fingers. Use your left foot as an anchor to stabilize the position, keeping your weight on the outer edge of your left foot and on the heel of your right foot. Use the pressure of your right shoulder or arm against your right knee to help keep your right knee in alignment with your right ankle and hip. This also helps you to open your chest, so that your left arm is able to point upward more easily.
   Hold this position for two or three breaths to find the relative ease in the position of the legs.
5. Inhaling, reach your left arm overhead to point toward the right side, with your palm facing down. Aim to create a straight line from the outside of your left foot to your left hand and fingertips.
   Sink further down into your hips if you can, to increase the stretch, without displacing the position of your legs. Open your left hip out and upward as much as possible (so that your entire torso aims to face the front). Your head and eyes look straight to the front; you can also turn your head and eyes to look up toward your left arm.

Timing: Hold for three to eight breaths, breathing into the open side of your chest. Keep your left leg extended to create a stable base. To recover, on an inhalation straighten your right leg slowly and reverse the path taken into the posture. Turn your feet so they are parallel and relax your arms at your sides for a few recovery breaths before repeating to the other side. After stretching both sides, move into a symmetrical counter-posture.

Option for hands

A. Place your hand on a block in front of your foot.

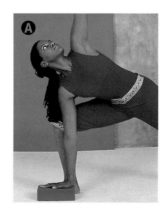

Extended version ☀☀☀

1. If you are comfortable in Utthita Parsvakonasana, place your left arm under your left thigh and your right arm behind your back.
2. Hold your left wrist in your right hand, keeping your left shoulder opened upward with your head and eyes looking upward.

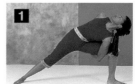

Cautions

• Only attempt this posture when you can comfortably hold Utthita Trikonasana.
• Take note of the cautions outlined for Utthita Trikonasana, taking care if you have a back or neck problem.
• Always follow the posture with a counter-posture.

• Take care not to strain – check that your breathing remains easy and that your facial muscles are not tense.
• If you feel any part of your body straining, inhale and slowly recover from the posture, either moving into the counter-posture or move into the Child's pose (p149), taking a few breaths to recover.

Summary: balancing postures

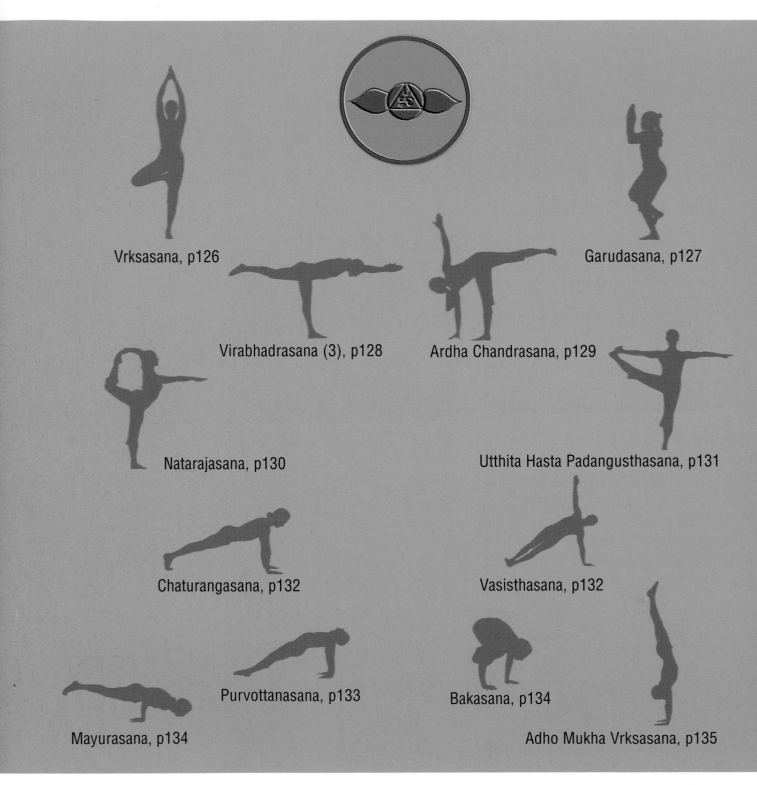

Vrksasana, p126

Garudasana, p127

Virabhadrasana (3), p128

Ardha Chandrasana, p129

Natarajasana, p130

Utthita Hasta Padangusthasana, p131

Chaturangasana, p132

Vasisthasana, p132

Purvottanasana, p133

Bakasana, p134

Mayurasana, p134

Adho Mukha Vrksasana, p135

BALANCING POSTURES
Standing and hand balances

Balance is a term often used to describe the attaining or maintaining of a position. It involves ease, poise and coordination through the equal or balanced use of the body. This could involve the balancing out of both sides of the body, or the finding of the central axis for balance when standing on one leg.

Balance is a dynamic activity of suspending the body in what merely looks like a static position. Every person possesses a natural sense of poise, which allows a posture to be maintained with ease and calmness. While balancing, your body should feel strong, centred and vitally alive, suffused with serenity; your mind should become ever more still, focused and peaceful.

A natural sense of balance

The body's natural, dynamic and oppositional stretch assists our sense of balance. In the upright position, this stretch comprises a downward, grounded feeling through the legs and feet. You should also feel an upward extension from the waist, as your spinal column lengthens and your head 'floats' on top of your shoulders.

In a one-legged balance, or a balance in a non-upright position, the oppositional stretch can occur between an arm and a leg in a side-to-side direction. It will help you to attain and maintain a balance if you keep an image of the counter-balance action in mind.

Willpower and concentration

Balances bring us up against our internal limitations and will-power, and are an excellent gauge of mental focus and concentration. Be gentle with yourself as you approach these often frustrating limitations, and by persevering you will strengthen your willpower and concentration. Rather than trying harder, practise with greater awareness so that you can let go of unnecessary tension and enter into a state of ease and centred balance, with breath flowing easily.

Balances are a good way to get to know how your mind can quite literally sway you off centre. They also offer an effective way to cultivate a state of inner stillness and serenity. Thus, these postures are an excellent training ground for the mental focus required for meditation.

Before you begin

- All standing balances start in Tadasana (p108), which establishes a stable and centred base.
- Keep your head centred and find a focus for your eyes at eye level, gently resting your eyes on that point and keeping your vision focused, throughout. Try closing your eyes or moving your focus around and see how much more difficult balance becomes.
- Be kind to yourself, especially in the beginning. Allow yourself to use the wall or a chair as a support to help you find your balance with greater ease.
- You should have three points of your feet firmly planted into the ground, with your toes spread out. Do not roll onto the outsides or insides of your feet or clench your toes.
- Remember to breathe to keep the posture alive.
- Feel the two-way extension of your body. This helps to distract the attention from the foot on which you are balancing and can help you keep centred.
- Take care not to strain in holding balances for too long. Rather hold them for a shorter period and perhaps repeat the balance after taking a few recovery breaths in a relaxed position, such as the Child's pose.
- A relaxed smile on your face will do wonders for your ability to ease into a balance.

VRKSASANA
The Tree
वृक्षासन

This pose gives an upward stretch to the body and is a good posture to use if you
are introducing your body to the art of balancing.

Timing: All the balances in this section are to be held for three to eight or even 16 breaths.
Breathing is mainly into the chest and ribcage area, with your shoulders relaxed and navel slightly pressed into your spine
to support your lower back (unless you are pregnant). Focus your attention on gently extending your spine and neck and
on a feeling of being grounded through your legs and feet. If you fall over, simply start again.
Hold asymmetrical balances for the same number of breaths on each side. After balancing on both sides,
move into a symmetrical rest pose, such as the Child's pose or Savasana, for a few recovery breaths.

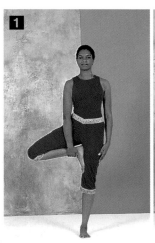 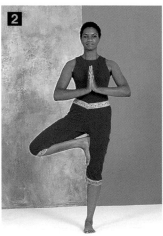 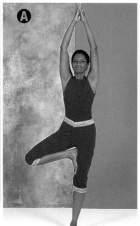 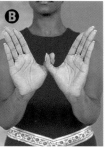 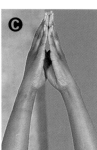

Vrksasana ☼ ☼ ☼

1. Bend your right knee, placing your heel as high up against
   the inside of your left leg as possible, aiming to place your
   right heel in your left groin (use your hands to help position
   your right foot). Your toes point downward, with knee and
   thigh opened out from the hip, so that your knee points out
   to the right side. Aim to keep your hips, torso and shoulders
   facing squarely to the front. Avoid sinking into the hip or
   raising your right hip.
2. Place your hands in the Prayer pose against your sternum.
   While holding this posture, feel the two-way stretch
   between your head and foot. Press your right foot against
   your left leg to help you hold the balance.
   After balancing on your left leg, return to Tadasana and
   repeat to the right.

Option for hands

A–C. Raise your hands in the Prayer pose above your head, so
that your fingers point upward. You will feel the two-way
stretch between your hands and your grounded foot.

Vrksasana in the Half Lotus ☼ ☼ ☼

1–2. Execute as for Vrksasana, with one leg in the Half Lotus.

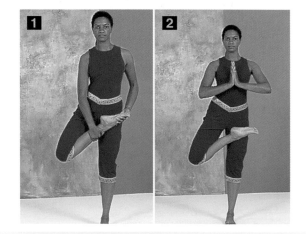

Benefits of all standing balances

- They tone and strengthen the muscles of the legs,
  knees, ankles and feet.
- They encourage the balanced development of the
  muscles of the torso, abdominals and back muscles.
- They encourage the stretching out of the spinal column.
- Hand balances tone and strengthen the muscles of the
  arms and shoulders.
- Hand balances strengthen and tone the abdominal and
  back muscles, and sometimes the leg muscles.

GARUDASANA
The Eagle

This posture is named after an eagle, which is considered to be the king of all birds.
Garuda is also the eagle deity in Indian mythology.

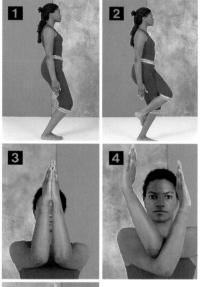

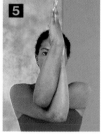

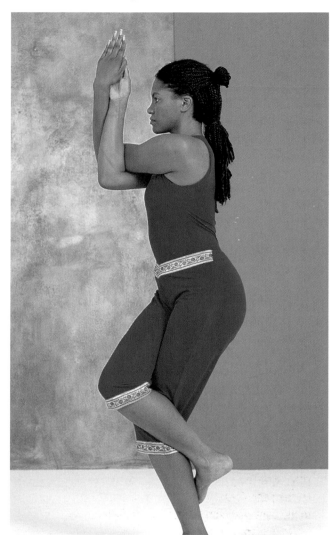

Garudasana ☀☀☀

1. Bend your knees slightly.
2. Bring your left leg to cross over your left, so that your thighs touch. Wrap your left foot around the back of your right leg (just under the calf or around the ankle).
3. Bend your elbows so that your forearms and hands stretch upward. Raise your elbows as close to shoulder height as you can.
4. Cross your left arm over your right, resting your left arm in the inside of your right elbow.
5. Move your right forearm back toward the right and cross it in front of your left forearm, which moves back toward the left. Touch palm to palm, keeping your fingers extended. Focus your eyes on your hands at eye level, while squeezing together your arms and legs.

Balance on your right foot, then return to Tadasana and repeat on the opposite side (see main photograph). Focus on keeping your arms and eye focus centred, your body upright and your knee facing the front. The two-way stretch is between head and grounded foot.

Option for hands

A. Join your hands, by holding your left thumb in your right hand and making fists with both hands.

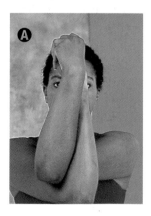

Cautions for all balances

- Balances can be strenuous and should be done with care, particularly if you suffer from high blood pressure or a heart condition.
- Always start with the simplest version of a balance.

- Hold a balance only for as long as you feel comfortable and remember to keep breathing to keep the balance vital and alive.
- If you are pregnant, do only the very simple balance postures, such as Vrksasana.

VIRABHADRASANA ✵✵✵
The Warrior
वृक्षासन

This is an extension of the Virabhadrasana postures, turning the posture into a balance on one leg, with arms, torso and raised leg forming a straight line parallel to the ground. Build the strength required for this posture by practising the first two versions of Virabhadrasana (pp114 & 116) and the back-bending postures such as the Locust (p88) and the Cobra (p86).

1. Assume the leg and foot position as for Virabhadrasana (1) (p114), with your left leg in front and bent to form a right angle; your thigh aiming to be parallel to the ground and your arms at your sides.

2. Inhaling, raise your arms and fingers forward and up, placing your arms next to your ears as you reach up through your fingers. Keep your head and eyes looking forward; head and neck remain in line with the rest of your spine. Shoulders are pressed down.

3. Exhaling, bend forward from your hips as you reach forward with your arms, bringing your torso and arms parallel to the ground. Keep your right leg extended with your foot well planted into the ground. Inhaling, feel the two-way stretch between your arms and right leg.

4. Exhaling and keeping your arms stretched forwards, shift your weight forwards over your left foot and leg, with your left knee still facing forward. Eyes look down to the ground or up toward your extended hands.

Raise your right leg, keeping it extended with toes pointing out behind you. Aim to bring your right leg parallel to the ground. Feel the two-way stretch between your fingers and the toes of your right foot.

(In the beginning, practice this Warrior posture holding onto the back of a chair or placing your hands against a wall.)

5–6. Balance in this position, or move on to extend your right leg on an exhalation while retaining the position of the rest of your body. Balance while focusing on the extension of the right leg and the two-way stretch between your fingers and your left foot. Stretch forward from your waist and backward with your raised leg.

Eyes focus down on the ground or toward your hands.

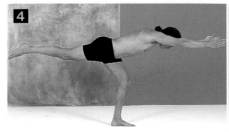

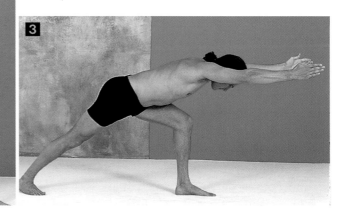

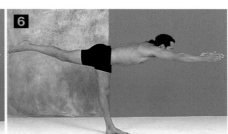

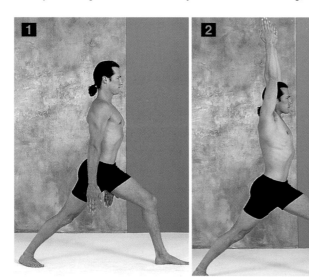

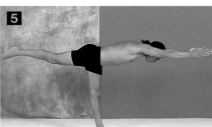

ARDHA CHANDRASANA ✷✷✷
The Half Moon

अर्ध चन्द्रासन

This posture resembles the shape of a half moon. It is an extension of Utthita Trikonasana and should only be attempted once Utthita Trikonasana and Utthita Parsvakonasana can be held comfortably.

1. Start by assuming Utthita Trikonasana (p118), bending to the right with the right knee bent and your right hand placed on the ground alongside your foot. Exhaling, shift your right arm to the side, cupping your hand and placing the fingertips on the ground a comfortable distance away from and slightly behind your leg. At the same time, shift your weight over your right foot, bringing your left foot slightly closer in to as you do so, using your right hand for support.

   Keep your left leg extended throughout. Either place your left hand at your side or keep it raised and extended vertically upwards as for Utthita Trikonasana. Eyes look down to your right hand to help you find your balance. If you struggle to reach the ground with your right hand, place your hand on a block (A).

2. Inhaling, keeping your left hip and shoulder open, rotate your torso to face the front. Exhaling, raise your left leg while simultaneously straightening your right leg. Find your balance over your right foot, using your right hand to support your balance.

   Open your left hip and shoulder by rotating your torso to the left. Rotate your right thigh outward, to avoid leaning back into your right leg. Aim to bring your left leg parallel to the ground, with your left leg rotated inward from the hip so that your knee faces forward.

3. Assist your balance by reaching up with your left arm and hand. If you feel stable in the position, raise your head and eyes to look up to your left hand. Balance in this position.

To recover, reverse your path as you return to the starting position. Return your feet to the centre and repeat the balance to the left. Then move into a symmetrical forward bend.

Practise Ardha Chandrasana against a wall initially to build confidence and find your alignment in the position.

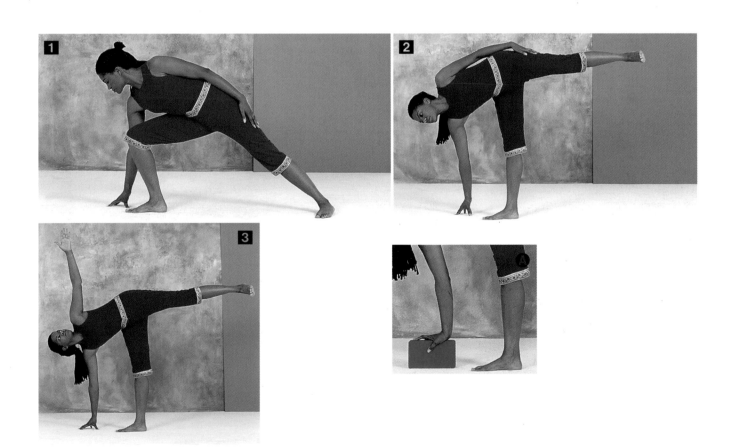

NATARAJASANA
The Dancer
नटराजासन

Nataraja is one of the many names given to Lord Shiva, who is known as the Lord of the Dance. To prepare for this posture, practice back bends, which in time will serve to build the necessary strength and flexibility required for Natarajasana. The simplified versions will also build up the strength and flexibility required for the full posture.

Preparation ☀☀

1. Start in Tadasana and raise your left arm so that it extends forward, at shoulder height, with palm facing down. Shift your weight onto your left leg, keeping your left knee pulled up into your thigh. Keep both knees touching as you bend your right leg backward from the knee, bringing your foot toward your buttocks. Hold of the outside of your right foot in your right hand. Balance, then return to Tadasana and repeat on the right leg.

Half Natarajasana ☀☀☀

2. Start as for the preparatory version, taking hold of the outside of your right ankle with your right hand.

   Raise your right leg as high as you can behind you, using your right hand to help you. Keep your raised leg behind you, with the front of your thigh facing down. Keep your right arm extended behind you, while your left arm extends forward at shoulder height (so that you feel a two-way stretch between your two arms in opposite directions).

   Balance in this position, then return to Tadasana and repeat on the opposite side.

Full Natarajasana ☀☀☀☀

3. Start as for the two preparatory versions. Rotate your right arm outward as you reach backward to take hold of your right big toe, between your index and second fingers or between your third and fourth fingers (whichever is more comfortable).

   Raise your right leg behind you, using your right arm and hand to help pull up your leg.

   As you raise the leg, rotate your right elbow inward so that it points upward and is brought in close to your ear. Aim to bring your right thigh parallel to the ground. Your left arm extends out in front of you, at shoulder height, with palm facing down.

   Balance in this position, then return slowly to Tadasana and repeat on the opposite side.

While balancing in Natarajasana, the focus for the two-way stretch is between your head and your grounded foot as well as between your two arms.

Keep your eyes looking out in front of you throughout.

Move into a symmetrical forward bend as a counter-posture, such as the Child's pose (p149).

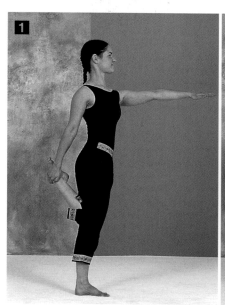
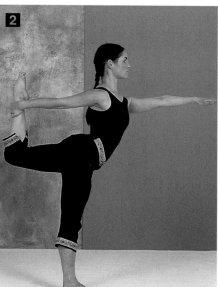
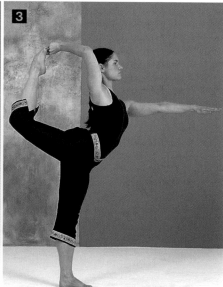

UTTHITA HASTA PADANGUSTHASANA
Balance posture
अत्थित हस्त पादाङ्गुष्ठासन

This posture is particularly effective for strengthening the legs and lower back.
Practise forward-bending postures, such as Janu Sirsasana (p70) to help build the strength to maintain the
alignment, particularly in the hips, required for Utthita Hasta Padangusthasana.

Preparation ☀☀

1. Start in Tadasana, placing your hands at your sides or on your hips with shoulder blades pulled together so that your chest is open.

   Inhaling, bend and raise your right knee in front of you, taking hold of the outside of your foot or your big toe between the thumb and first two fingers of your right hand. Use your hand to draw your foot as close as you can into your groin, with your knee pointing out in front of you. Pull back slightly in your right hip to keep your hips squarely facing the front.

   Balance in this position, then return to Tadasana and repeat the balance on the opposite side.

Utthita Hasta Padangusthasana ☀☀☀

1–2. Start as for the preparatory version, extending your right leg, still holding the foot or big toe. Pull back slightly in your right hip and shoulder to keep your hips and shoulders facing the front. If you wish to increase this stretch, keep your spine and legs extended and bring your raised leg up toward your chest and your torso down toward your raised leg.

Balance in this position. Then return to Tadasana and repeat the balance on your right leg (raising your left leg). The focus of attention is on the stretch between your head and grounded foot. Focus on keeping your right hip and shoulder back while your right leg is extended.

Option

To help you feel the alignment of your hips and find your balance in this position, practise this posture with your raised leg placed on a ledge in front of you.

Version with leg to the side ☀☀☀

3. Execute as for Utthita Hasta Padangusthasana, raising your right leg with your knee and thigh turned out to the right side. You can hold your foot or your big toe. Try to keep your hips level and square to the front and your torso centred (avoid leaning away from your raised leg and also avoid leaning forwards or backward).

   Once you find your balance, extend your left arm to the left side, so that your arms are parallel to the ground. You can also try this version resting your leg on a ledge, before moving on to the unsupported version.

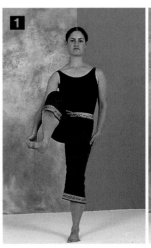
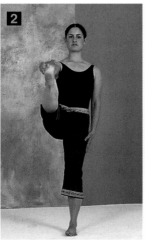
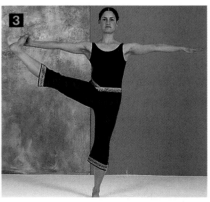

HAND BALANCES
नटराजासन

These hand balances require – and build – strength in the upper body and arms. Start by doing the simplest of the postures, which will help you build the wrist, forearm, upper arm and shoulder strength necessary for the more complex balances. Hand balances are also excellent for toning and strengthening the muscles of the abdomen and back. Take care to work only with the versions you can comfortably execute, and do not strain yourself in holding the postures for too long.

Timing: All balances are to be held for three to eight breaths, or longer if you can. If the posture is asymmetrical, take care to hold the balance for the same number of breaths on both sides.

CHATURANGASANA ✸✸
The Plank

A. Start on all fours, with hands under shoulders and knees under hips. Curl your toes under and straighten your legs, reaching one leg at a time out behind you. Maintain a feeling of lifting out of your shoulders.

Hold your body in a straight line. Avoid dipping your hips out of line with the rest of your body, as this may strain your lower back. Eye focus is down to the ground between or just beyond your hands.

The two-way oppositional stretch can be felt through the crown of the head and the heels as you hold this balance.

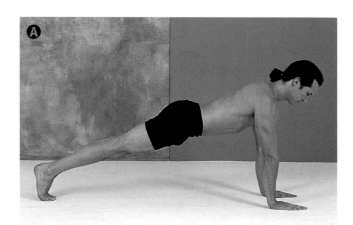

VASISTHASANA ✸✸
The Inclined Plank
वसिष्ठासन

B. Start in the Plank and rotate your entire body to the left, so that the weight of your body is supported entirely on the outer side of your left foot and your body is facing the front.

Raise your right arm, extending the arm, hand and fingers vertically upward. Keep your torso and hips in line with your legs – don't allow them to dip. It is helpful to rotate the top of the left arm forward as you reach through your right arm, to give a feeling of 'lifting out' of the left shoulder. Keep head and eyes looking forward. (This posture can also be done with your right arm held at your side.)

Balance, move back into the Plank, then move into Vasisthasana, balancing on your opposite side. After balancing on both sides, move into the Child's pose (p149) for a few recovery breaths.

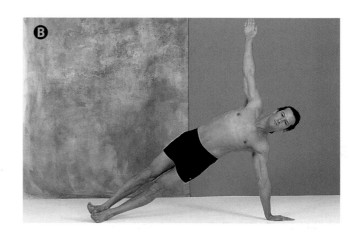

Version with leg balance ✳✳✳

C. Start as for the Inclined Plank, bending your right knee, opening it out to face upward. Take hold of your right foot or big toe between the thumb and first two fingers of your right hand, placing your right arm in front of your right leg. Then straighten your right leg upward as you straighten your arm, which holds the toe. Turn your head to look up toward your right hand. Your arm and leg should have a feeling of pulling upward.

Balance in this position, then return to the Plank and repeat to the other side.

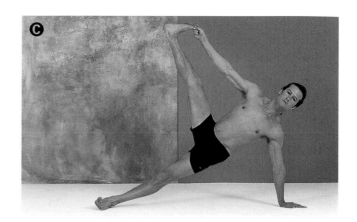

PURVOTTANASANA ✳✳✳
The Inclined Plank in a back bend

'Purva' means 'east' and refers to the front of the body. 'Purvotta' refers to an intense stretch of the front of the body. Do not do this posture if you have a neck problem.

1. Start sitting with your legs outstretched and held together in front of you. Rest your arms behind you, with your fingers pointing out behind you or in toward you. Take a few deep breaths into your chest before moving into the posture.

2. Inhaling deeply into your chest, raise your hips and chest as high as you can, while keeping your legs extended and your feet as flat on the ground as possible. Allow your head to drop backward.

Balance, then slowly return to the sitting position and rest for a few recovery breaths, hanging forward over your legs (as for a relaxed version of Pascimottanasana) or in the Child's pose. This posture can be used as a back bend and as a counter-posture for forward bends.

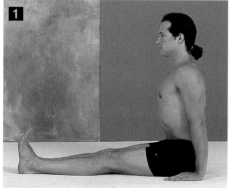

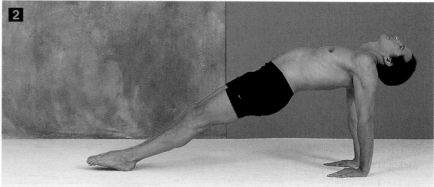

Extended versions ✳✳✳

A. Start as for the above version and raise one leg off the ground. Balance, while keeping both legs extended. Repeat, raising the other leg.

B. Start as for the above version with both feet on the ground and raise one arm vertically upward. Balance, then repeat, raising the other arm.

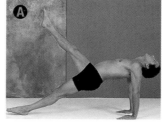

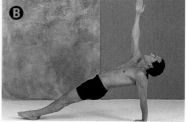

BAKASANA ✹✹✹
The Crow
बकासन

'Baka' translates as 'crow', although this posture is also sometimes known as Kakasana, the Crane.

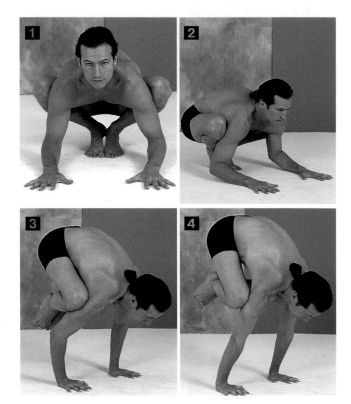

1. Squat with your feet together and your knees opened out to the sides. Place your hands flat on the ground in front of you, spreading your fingers. Your elbows are bent and your torso leans forward. Eyes look down to the ground, finding a point of focus to assist your balance.
2. Lean further forward as you raise your heels off the ground so that you can rest your shins on the backs of your upper arms as near to your armpits as possible.
3. Raise your feet off the ground toward your buttocks as you lean your weight into your arms and hands, keeping your arms bent. Round your spine as you do so by contracting your abdominal muscles and keeping your legs well tucked in. This will help you to achieve a feeling of lightness in the position. Raise your head slightly to look out in front of you, to help counteract the tendency to fall forwards in the position.
4. If you can, straighten your arms in the balance. Hold the balance. To recover, return to the squat position and relax in the Child's pose or the Corpse pose (p148) for a few recovery breaths.

MAYURASANA ✹✹✹
The Peacock
मयूरासन

'Mayura' means 'peacock'. In its advanced form, this posture resembles a peacock with its feathers displayed. Most practitioners find this posture more strenuous than the Crow, as it is the abdomen that rests into the arms.

1. Kneel on your haunches and place your hands together, flat on the ground, with your fingers facing in and forearms facing the front. Hold your elbows close together.
2. Bend your elbows as you lean forward, resting your abdomen on your elbows.
3. With care, lean further forward, so that your weight is centred over your hands, with toes curled under you.

4. Shift your weight forward over your hands so that your feet rise behind you. Do not try to raise your legs off the ground, as your weight may not be centred correctly over your hands. Keep your legs straight and parallel to the ground.
   Balance, breathing gently. The pressure of your elbows in your abdomen gives a strong massage to the abdominal area, benefiting digestion. To recover, reverse your path, moving slowly and with care.

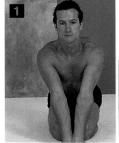
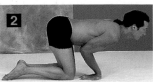
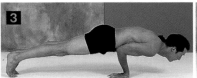
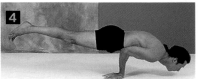

The Peacock: extended version ☀☀☀☀

A. Move into Mayurasana. Raise your legs up as high as you can, while either keeping your head on the ground or allowing your chin to extend down toward the ground. Keep your legs in line with your spine as you do so, so that your body forms one straight line.

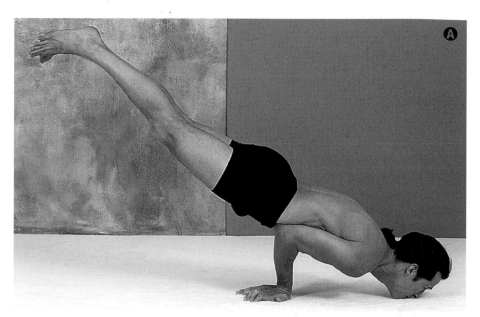

ADHO MUKHA VRKSASANA
The Hand Stand
अध्यो मुख वृक्षासन

'Adho Mukha' means 'face-down' and a 'vrksasana' is a tree – this posture is like an upside-down tree. It requires strong arm and shoulder muscles and should be practiced with care. Practise Adho Mukha Svanasana (the Downward-facing Dog Stretch, p94) to build up the strength in your arms. Remember that this is an inverted posture, so do not do the Hand Stand if you suffer from a heart condition, high blood pressure or any eye condition that does not allow for inversion.

Hand Stand against a wall ☀☀☀

1. Stand facing a wall. Place your hands on the ground, shoulder-width apart, with fingers pointing toward the wall. Straighten your elbows and walk your feet toward your hands.

2. On an exhalation, jump one leg up against the wall and then raise the other, so that both feet rest against the wall.

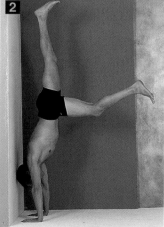

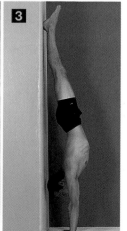

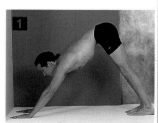

3. Reach up out of your shoulders, so that your arms are extended and your hands push down into the ground. Hold your legs together and parallel. Your eyes look in front of you or to your hands.

Balance in this position, with weight equally distributed on both hands. The two-way stretch can be felt between your feet and your hands.

Hand Stand away from a wall ☀☀☀☀

Very advanced practitioners can also practice jumping both legs up into the handstand at the same time (i.e. holding your legs together from the beginning).

Summary: inverted postures

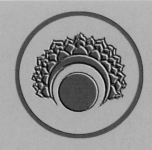

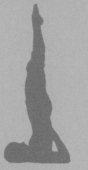

Sarvangasana, p138

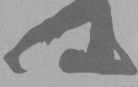

Halasana, p140

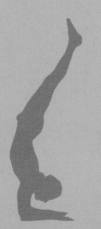

Vrscikasana, p145

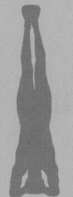

Salamba Sirsasana, p142

Timing for inverted postures: Hold each posture for three to 16 breaths or longer if you can comfortably do so.
Counter-postures: After practising any of these postures, move into the counter-posture suggested. Thereafter, it is beneficial to move into Tadasana for a few breaths and then relax in Savasana (p148). This will help the blood circulation return to normal after inversion.

Cautions

There are certain conditions in which inversion is contra-indicated. If you are in doubt about a condition you may have, consult your doctor or health practitioner before attempting inverted postures.

Do not attempt inverted postures if:
- you suffer from a heart condition
- you have high blood pressure (even when controlled by medication)
- you have an eye problem, such as a detached retina

INVERTED POSTURES

It is quite common to see children at playgrounds jumping, tumbling, hanging upside down and doing cartwheels. This renders them healthy and energetic, as their blood circulation, co-ordination and balance are constantly being moved about and challenged.

As we grow older, we tend to become less active, which is a common contributing factor to poorer blood circulation, reduced energy levels and loss of youthfulness. Yoga offers one way to keep twisting, bending and inverting your body and exercising your heart and all other muscles in your body.

Inverted postures are an indispensable part of a Yoga practice. They influence the functioning of the body in numerous ways; benefits are experienced on a physiological, mental and spiritual level, and these postures revitalize the entire system. They can help alleviate fatigue, insomnia, headaches, varicose veins, digestive problems and excess tension and anxiety, for example. Some practitioners go so far as to describe these inverted postures, particularly Sirsasana (the Headstand), as a panacea for all who practise.

The immune system

On a physiological level, inverted postures enhance the functioning of the immune system. Many people suffer from poor blood circulation, which results in the tissues of the body not being sufficiently nourished and revitalized. Inverted postures enhance blood circulation throughout the body, helping to nourish those deprived tissues and tone the endocrine system.

Inverted postures also give the digestive system a well-deserved rest, allowing the abdominal muscles and viscera to regain their tone. Thus, by inverting the body, internal organs that may have become sluggish are activated. Inverting the body also gives a well-deserved rest, in the anti-gravity position, to the heart.

Alleviating tension

Inverted postures help to counteract and alleviate bodily tension. Holding excess tension in the body can restrict blood circulation. In the anti-gravity position, the entire body (and particularly the torso) can easily find a state of relaxation.

These postures also help to counteract the pull of gravity in the process of ageing. By helping to keep the spine lengthened and elastic, they allow the spinal fluid and the nerves that stem from the spine to continue to flow or communicate freely and therefore easily nourish and energize the entire body well into old age.

The increased blood supply to the facial tissues also helps to reduce or even prevent wrinkles on the face.

Rejuvenating the brain

The increased blood supply to the brain can rejuvenate that organ's cells and enhance all mental faculties, including memory and motor skills. In addition, inverted postures enhance concentration and develop the practitioner's willpower, thus enhancing meditation practice.

The pineal and pituitary glands

On a subtle level, inverted postures work mainly on the Sahasrara chakra – the crown energy centre. This energy centre is associated with the pineal gland, situated in the head. This gland is referred to as the third eye and is associated with higher states of consciousness or awareness.

The pituitary gland is nourished in inverted postures – it is known as 'the Master gland', as it regulates the functioning of all the glands in the body.

In the Head Stand, the main beneficiaries are the pineal and the pituitary glands. In the Shoulder Stand, the blood supply and nourishment is focused on the thyroid gland in the throat area, which regulates metabolism.

- you have an ear problem where inversion is not advised
- you are pregnant. Only do inverted postures if you are well practised in them, and even so, preferably practise against a wall or using a chair for support. Avoid inversion in the last trimester of pregnancy

- if you are menstruating
- If you develop any pain or discomfort in your neck or anywhere else in your body. Often injuries occur only when your body is not held in correct alignment. Consult your Yoga teacher before continuing to practise.

SARVANGASANA
The Shoulder Stand
सर्वांगासन (सालम्ब सर्वांगासन)

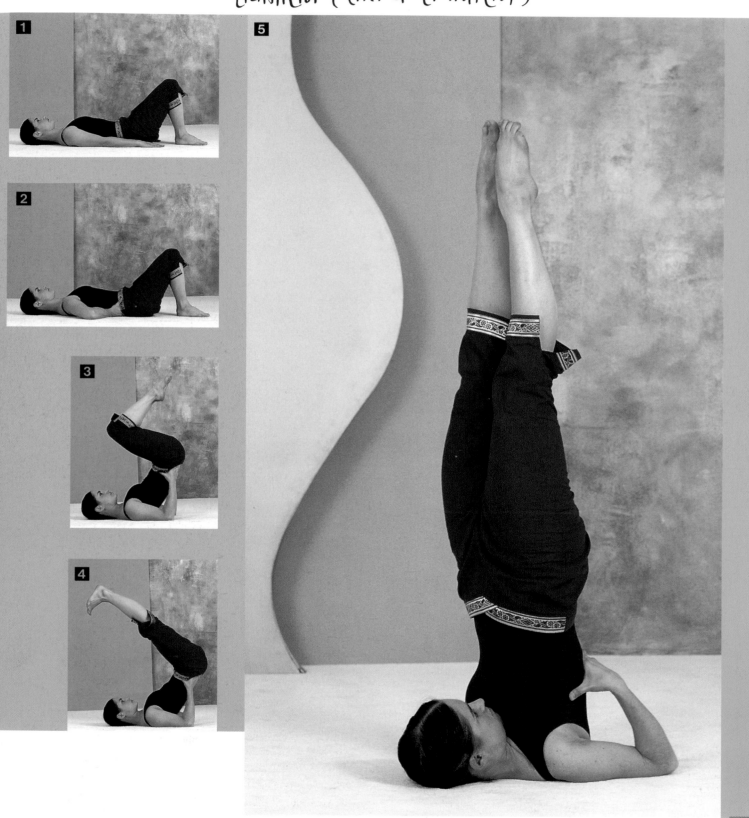

This posture may also be called Salamba Sarvangasana – 'salamba' means 'supported' and 'sarvanga' means 'whole' or 'everything' and refers to the benefits yielded by this posture to all parts of the body. 'Salamba' also refers to a neck balance. This posture works on the Visuddha chakra (the throat energy centre) and nourishes the brain with an increased blood supply. Prepare for Sarvangasana with leg raises and Setu Bandha Sarvangasana (p99). Never turn your head out of alignment in the Shoulder Stand. If you experience discomfort in any area of your body, move out of the posture into a rest pose.

Preparation: Viparita Karani ☀☀

1. Lie on your back and bend your knees, placing the soles of your feet on the ground, with your legs held together.
2. Place your hands on your waist, with thumbs on the sides of your waist and palms and fingers supporting underneath your back.
3. Exhaling, swing your knees up over your abdomen, keeping your legs bent and raising your torso. Use your hands as support for your back, while pressing your elbows into the ground. Bring your elbows as close together as you can, taking care to keep your hands level.
4. Straighten your legs with legs and feet pointing diagonally upwards. Balance in this relaxed position. To recover, use your hands to support your back as you gently lower your torso.

Sarvangasana ☀☀☀

1–4. Start as for Viparita Karani.
5. Inhaling, push your hips further forward as you bring your chest toward your chin and aim your legs and torso toward the vertical. Bring your elbows closer together and shift your hands to your upper back.
Find the relaxation in the posture, keeping your feet relaxed or extended, your head centred and neck relaxed. While holding the posture, keep your body extended from your chest up to your feet. Hold your legs together throughout. Breathe easily.

To recover, use your arms to support your back as you slowly return to the starting position lying on your back. Then move into a counter-pose such as the Fish (p92), which opens up the throat and chest area. You can also move straight from the Shoulder Stand into the Plough (p140), before moving into a counter-posture.

Preparation: Sarvangasana against a wall ☀

1. Lie on your back, with your hips a small distance away from a wall, so your feet rest against the wall, with your legs at a slight angle to your body. Bend your knees and place the soles of your feet against the wall, keeping your legs parallel and hip distance apart.
2. Walk your feet up the wall as you push forward in your lower back and hips.
3. At the highest point, your chest presses against your chin. This supported version can be practised on its own or used as a preparation for Sarvangasana.

Option: lying on a blanket

A. A blanket provides a soft surface for you to lie on and slightly raises your shoulders off the ground.

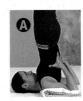

Viparita Karani as a rest pose

1–2. Lie against a wall, placing a folded blanket/s under your hips and resting your legs up against the wall. Allow your arms to rest on the ground behind your head. This version offers a wonderful relaxation for the legs and is beneficial for leg problems, such as varicose veins, or to relax your legs after a Yoga session or when you have been on your feet all day.

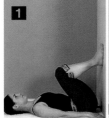
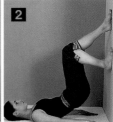
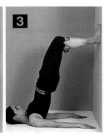
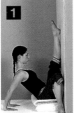
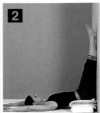

HALASANA
The Plough
हलासन

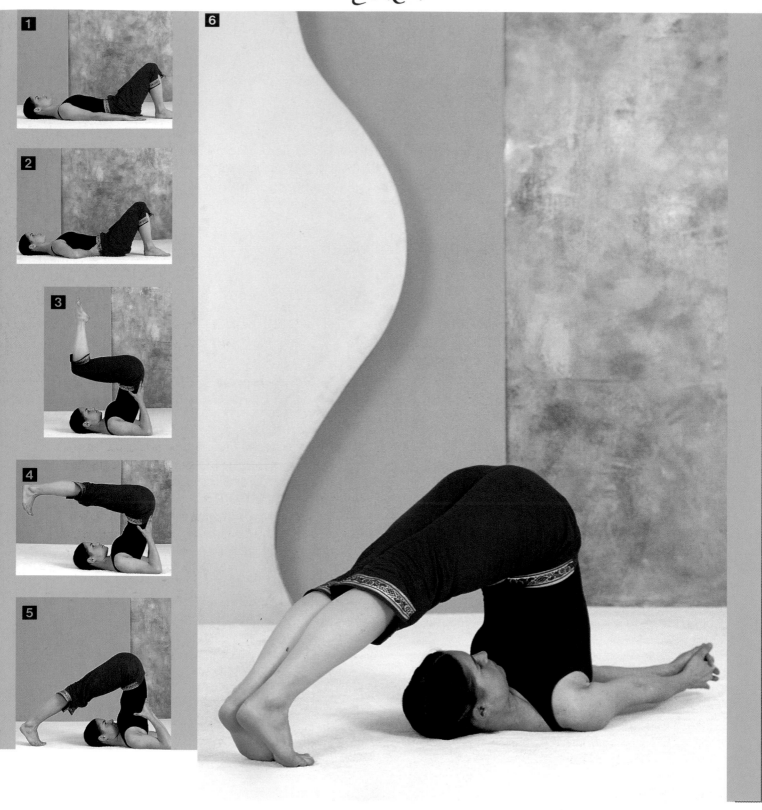

'Hala' means 'plough'. This posture 'ploughs' our blood supply and energies into our head area, availing this energy for higher mental and spiritual work. In Halasana, the brain and nervous system are able to relax. This posture works on the Visuddha chakra (the throat energy centre), as well as nourishing the brain with an increased blood supply. It stretches the entire spinal column, offering relief from spinal tension or problems. It should always be practised with care. Prepare for Halasana with leg raises and Setu Bandha Sarvangasana (p99).

Preparation: Ardha Halasana ☀☀

1. Start as for Sarvangasana on your back, with knees bent and the soles of your feet on the ground.
2. Place your hands behind your waist as for Sarvangasana.
3. Round your spine as you raise your hips off the ground, bringing your knees and thighs over your abdomen.
4. Straighten your legs so that they are parallel to the ground. Press your elbows to the ground to help move your hips over your shoulders and bring your chest in toward your chin. Feet are relaxed or extended.

Halasana ☀☀☀

5. Execute as for Ardha Halasana, bringing your toes down to touch the ground, while keeping your legs extended.
6. If you are comfortable in this position, extend your arms, palms down on the ground behind you, or clasping your hands; alternatively, place your arms on the ground behind your head. Find the relaxation in the posture. Take care to keep your head and neck centred throughout.

To recover, slowly bend your knees and support your spine with your hands, as you reverse the path taken into the posture, return to the starting position lying on your back. Move into the Fish as a counter-posture or any other simple back bend that gives a stretch to the throat and chest area.

Option: lying on a blanket

A. A blanket provides a soft surface for you to lie on and slightly raises your shoulders off the ground.

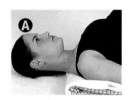

Ardha Halasana as a rest pose

B. A relaxed version can be done with legs resting on a chair. Relax your arms on the ground behind your head.

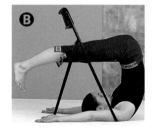

Karnapidasana (the Spider) ☀☀☀

A. Execute as for Halasana, bending your knees toward the ground next to your ears. Hug your arms around your legs for support. This posture gives an extended stretch to the lumbar spine. If your neck feels strained, try keeping your hands on your back for support, while relaxing your knees down toward your ears.

Option for hands

B. Take hold of your heels or calves with your hands.

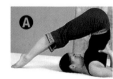
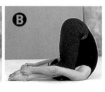

Extended options ☀☀☀

A. Point your feet.
B. Spread your legs apart and curl your toes under on the ground; extend your arms to your sides, higher than the line of your shoulders, and take hold of your big toes.
C. With your hands supporting your back, walk your feet to the right, until your hips and lower back twist and your feet are to the right of your shoulder. Keep your spine centred. Hold for equal time on both sides, then move into Halasana or Karnapidasana to restore symmetry to your body.

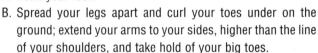
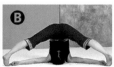
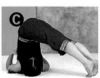

SALAMBA SIRSASANA
The Head Stand

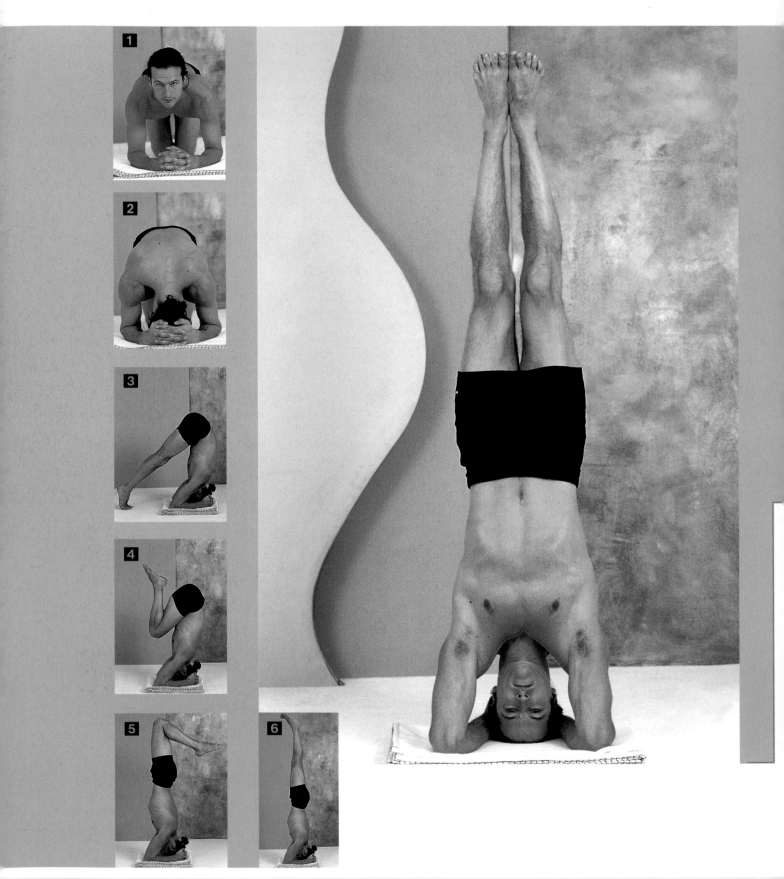

'Salamba' means 'supported' and 'Sirsa' refers to the head. This posture is often referred to as the king of all postures, because it nourishes the brain. If you have a neck problem, either do not do the Head Stand or do Sasamgasana, with your hands used for support. For all the versions of the Head Stand below, place a folded blanket or flat cushion under your head so that your head rests on a soft yet supportive surface.

Preparation for Sirsasana ☀☀☀

1. Start on all fours, sitting back toward your heels. Clasp your fingers, placing hands and elbows on the ground in front of you, with your palms facing toward you and your elbows apart and resting on the ground.
2. Place the crown of your head on the ground, up close against your hands.
3. Curl your toes under and straighten your legs. Walk your feet in toward you, until your torso and hips are raised vertically upwards. Hold your abdominal muscles contracted as you pull back in your hips.

   If you are comfortable in this position, move onto the next position, otherwise practise holding in this position in preparation for the Full Head Stand.
4. Bend your knees and raise your legs so that your thighs rest over your abdomen as you bring your torso into a vertical position. Hold your legs together throughout and balance on your head and forearms.

   Keep a feeling of lifting up and out of your shoulders.

   If you are comfortable in this position, move on to the next stage; otherwise hold this position.
5. Raise and pull back your knees as you push forwards in your hips, so that your thighs are brought in line with your torso, with your knees pointing upward and your feet lowered behind you.
6. Extend your legs, bringing your entire body into a vertical line. Your feet can be relaxed or extended.

   You can also practise the Head Stand against a wall for support, then graduate to a small distance away from the wall, so you can use the wall only if you need to.

   Eventually, move into the centre of the room.

Timing: Hold for three to six breaths, or longer.
To recover, reverse your path slowly and carefully, then move into the Child's pose, with your head resting on two fists, so that your head and neck are supported in line with the rest of your spine. Take a few recovery breaths in this position before slowly recovering to the upright position.

Option for arms

1. Place your hands flat on the ground, slightly in front of you, with fingers inward and arms shoulder-width apart.
2. Your hands support your head stand, with elbows raised and upper arms held parallel to the ground.

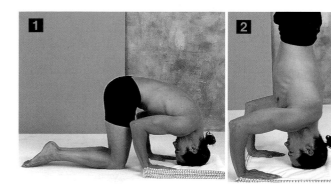

Preparation: Sasamgasana (the Hare) ☀☀

1. Start in the Child's pose, placing your hands and forearms (palms down) onto the ground, so that your hands are in line with your ears.
2. Pushing gently from your lower spine, roll up onto the crown of your head, using your arms for support, so that there is no pressure on your neck. Hold.
3. If you do not have a neck problem, clasp your hands, palm to palm, behind your back as you extend your arms upward. Support this position by contracting your abdominal muscles and rounding your spine. Hold.

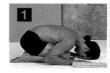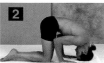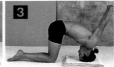

Extended versions in Sirsasana ☀ ☀ ☀ ☀

Try some of these variations of Sirsasana, holding for three to six breaths, holding asymmetrical positions for an equal length of time on each side:

A. Walk one leg forward and the other backward, in a scissor-like motion. Hold, then change legs.

B. Bend your knees, opening them out to the sides and pressing the soles of your feet together.

C. Spread your legs apart sideways, flexing your feet and reaching out through your heels.

D. Keeping your legs together, bring them half way down to the ground, so that your legs are held parallel to the ground, with feet flexed.

E. Lower one leg to the ground in front of you, in line with your hip. Hold, then repeat with your other leg.

F. Keeping both legs raised, revolve your torso and legs from the waist, holding to one side and then to the other.

G. Twist from your waist as you extend your legs away from each other in the scissor-like motion. Hold, then repeat to the other side.

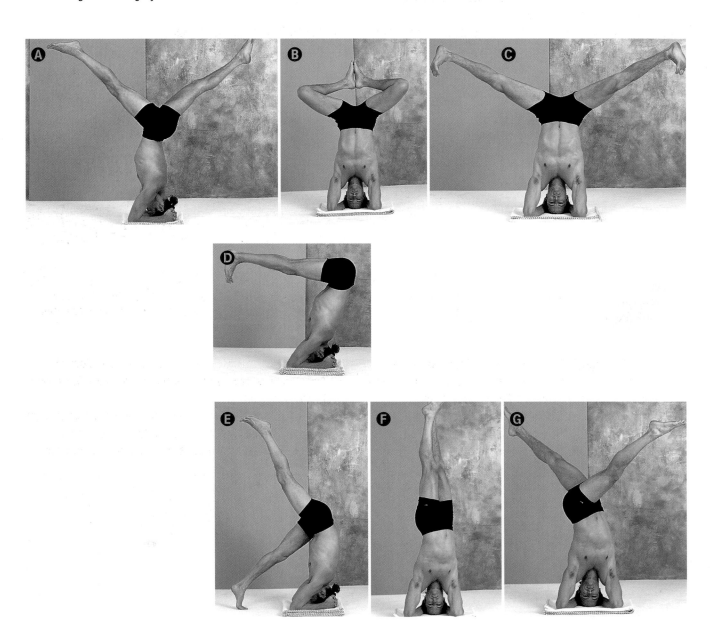

VRSCIKASANA
The Scorpion
तृश्चिकासन

'Vrscika' is a scorpion. This pose in its advanced stage resembles a scorpion with its tail arched back over its head. Vrscikasana is also known as Pinca Mayurasana, the tail feather of a peacock. It requires strength in the shoulders and upper back, although when in the position, little strength is needed as you find your balance and relaxation into the posture. Practise the Head Stand first and when you can hold it comfortably for at least six breaths, then move on to attempt Vrscikasana.

Preparation: Vrscikasana against a wall ☀ ☀ ☀

1. Start on all fours, a small distance from a wall. Place your forearms and hands on the ground, shoulder-width apart and on a folded blanket. Begin with your head placed between your arms on the ground.
2–3. Walk your feet in toward the wall. Then, one leg at a time, place your feet or heels against the wall.

4. Push your hips slightly forward and tighten your buttock for support. Your eyes look down to your hands or out beyond your hands. Feel lifted out of your shoulders throughout.

Vrscikasana ☀ ☀ ☀ ☀
Execute as for the preparation, away from a wall.

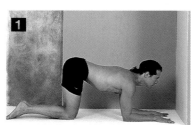
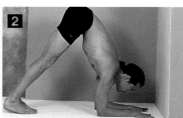
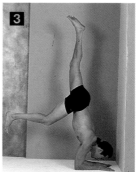
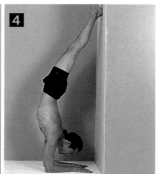

Timing: Hold for three to six breaths, or longer.
To recover, reverse the path taken into the posture, keeping your head raised, until moving into a counter-posture such as the Child's pose. Rest for a few recovery breaths in the Child's pose, with your head on two fists.

Dynamic preparation to build strength

1. Place your forearms on the ground, with your elbows shoulder-width apart and your fingers interlocked.
2. Move into the Downward-facing Dog Stretch. Reach forwards with the crown of your head.
3. Inhaling, lower your hips, bringing them in line with your torso and legs (into the Plank, resting on your elbows).
As you exhale, raise your hips and return to the Downward-facing Dog Stretch.
Move between the Dog Stretch and the Plank four to eight times, co-ordinating your breath with the movement.
You can also hold each position for three to six breaths.

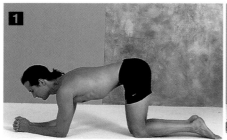
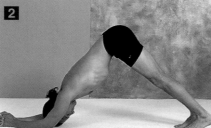
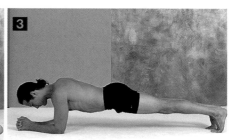

Summary: rest and relaxation postures

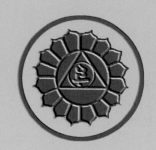

Savasana, p148

Supta Vajrasana, p149

Apanasana, p149

REST AND RELAXATION POSTURES

The greatest power in efficient and effective movement is when the ability to relax is also present.

A cat is the perfect example – when it has its eyes on a bird or mouse, it waits in repose, seemingly motionless, easy and graceful with no muscular tension; instead, it has an intense vitality, focus and readiness for action. There are no quivering muscles, no nerves 'on edge', no fidgeting, no perspiration; there is no strain in the waiting, no wasteful motion or muscular tension. And when the moment of action arrives, within an instant, energy surges into fresh muscles and calm nerves, to create a spectacular leap.

A state of readiness

Relaxation practice can be seen as a way in which to cultivate a state of readiness and vitality, which is the inherent potential of relaxed muscles and nerves.

This, coupled with meditation practice (which trains the calm, unwavering focus of attention and intention) and a stretch and strength programme (such as Hatha Yoga) that tones the physical body, can set free the greatness and power of human potential.

The use of rest postures

The rest poses are not graded as for the other postures. They are all suitable for everyone, with one or two exceptions, where small adaptations may be required.

All the rest poses presented in this section are symmetrical and help to restore a state of balance in the body.

Rest poses are recommended at the end and sometimes also at the beginning of a session.

They are also recommended at various stages during a session, to allow the body to rest between postures, and can be used as counter-postures to back bends, side bends or twists.

The rest pose particularly recommended for the end and for the beginning of a session is Savasana (the Corpse pose).

SAVASANA
The Corpse pose
शवासन

This is the most basic of the relaxation postures. It involves lying on your back, with legs straight and slightly apart; the feet and legs are relaxed, with the arms held, palms up, at a 45° angle to the torso. The back of the neck is extended so that your spine is lengthened, with your chin tucked in toward your chest. Savasana restores symmetry in your body. Take care that you are truly lying straight and evenly relaxed on the right and left sides.

To help your body let go of tension, work from feet to face and head, progressively tensing each muscle or muscle group, holding it tense for a few moments and then letting go, imagining that with each letting go the respective area sinks heavily into the ground, allowing all tension to melt down into the earth.

Stretch your legs away from you by flexing your feet and reaching forward with your heels. Then allow your legs to relax. This allows the surface underneath your legs to make greater contact with the ground.

You can do the same with your arms if you wish, by extending them away from you and then letting them relax into the ground. To further relax your abdominal area, spread your legs further apart, allowing them to flop open. Check that your breathing is easy, with a natural flow.

- Cover your eyes with a piece of clothing or a cloth.
- Place a cushion or folded blanket under your head for greater comfort.

- Let your mind scan your body while you lie relaxed, to check for any areas that may require a little extra attention to truly let go and relax – invite these areas to let go, and allow them to feel supported by the ground.
- Perhaps take a few breaths, concentrating your attention on the respective area.
- It may help to imagine yourself lying in a beautiful meadow or on a cloud or on warm sand on a beach, with the sound of the sea in the distance or any other image that helps you to feel soothed and relaxed.

Remain in Savasana for about five minutes.

Savasana before the session allows you to let go of the tensions of the day or night before moving on to the practice of postures.

After the practice, Savasana allows you to fully absorb the energy that has been released and accumulated throughout the Yoga session.

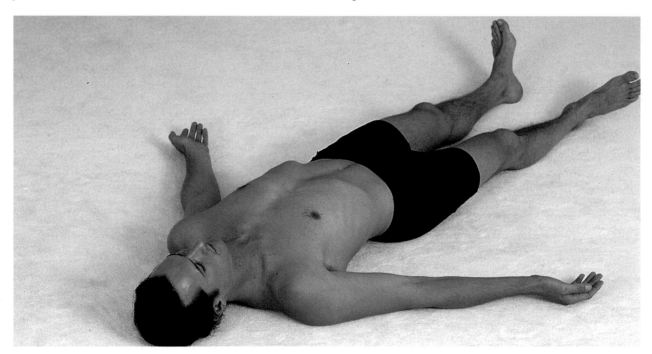

To come out of Savasana without disturbing your peace, stretch out your body and take a deep breath (yawn if you can). Roll onto your side into the foetal position, then gradually ease your way up to a sitting or standing position, moving slowly without any sudden or jerky movements.

SUPTA VAJRASANA
The Child's pose
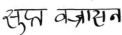

The Child's pose can also be regarded as a version of Vajrasana. In this pose, the body is held in the position of a foetus in the womb, which has a soothing effect on body and mind alike. It involves a forward bend of the torso and allows the entire spinal column to relax, particularly in the lumbar region, and has a calming effect on the nervous system.

A. Sit on your haunches, with your arms relaxed at your sides. Sit back onto your heels and bend forwards, placing your forehead on the ground. Your arms rest at your sides alongside your body, with shoulders relaxed over your knees.

Option for hands

B. If you have high blood pressure, a heart condition or any eye problem in which the head should remain above the level of the heart, place one fist on top of the other and rest your forehead on your two fists.

Another option is to relax your arms at your sides and place your head on a cushion or pile of books, so that your head is supported in line with the rest of your spine.

If you are pregnant, spread your knees apart.

Caution

If you have varicose veins or problems with your knees, rather do Savasana or Apanasana.

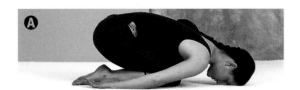

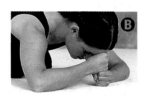

APANASANA
The Wind-relieving position

This position is particularly beneficial for digestion. It also gives a wonderful massage to the lower back and can help to relieve tension in the area. Apanasana can be used as a soothing counter-posture to back bends and spinal twists, as well as postures requiring strong work with your legs, such as standing postures and balances. It can also function as a posture in its own right, and can be executed dynamically or statically.

Lie on your back, with your body straight and chin slightly tucked in, so that the back of your neck is long. Bend both legs, hugging your knees in over your abdomen with your arms. Keep your lower spine (all the way to the coccyx) in contact with the ground.

Option for legs

A. Open your knees to work on mobility and flexibility in the hip joint. (If you are pregnant, this version helps to mobilize the hips in preparation for childbirth.)

If your knees are parallel, the position works more on the lower abdominal and lower back area.

Static version

Hold the pose for three to eight breaths, or longer.

Dynamic version

1. Hold your knees with your hands, keeping your legs together and over your abdomen.
2. Inhaling, release your knees as far away from you as your arms will allow. Exhaling, ease your knees back over your abdomen. Repeat three to eight times, feeling the massage to the lower back area.

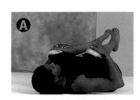

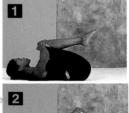

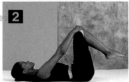

Benefits

- Gives a gentle massage to the abdominal organs, thus aiding digestion, relieving wind or gas.
- Tones the abdominal organs.
- Gently stretches out the lower back.

CHAPTER 6

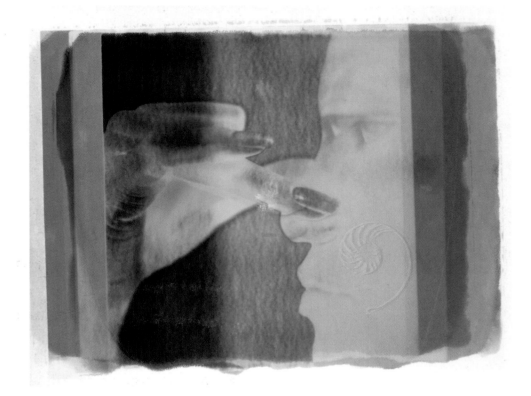

BREATHING

Cautions

There are certain conditions in which Pranayama is contra-indicated:

- if you have a migraine
- if you suffer from epilepsy
- if you are recovering from abdominal surgery
- if you have any medical condition for which you are on medication or are in the process of recovery.

Avoid deep inhalations if:

- you have a heart condition or problem
- you have high blood pressure (hypertension)

Avoid deep exhalations if:

- you have low blood pressure (hypotension)
- you suffer from depression.

If you have hypoglycaemia, do only calm, simple breathing exercises.

PRANAYAMA
The art of breath control

'Prana' means 'life force' and 'ayama' means 'to lengthen'. Pranayama, therefore, is the art of lengthening the breath and, through the breath, enhancing the life force and energy within us. The breath is the link between the mind and the body, and through the breath we take in Prana, the subtle life force that animates all living things.
Pranayama is a means of purifying the physical and subtle body through the breath. It calms the nervous system, focusing and quieting the mind and cultivating a feeling of spaciousness and serenity in body and mind.
Pranayama practised before meditation will greatly assist your Yoga practice, as it creates an environment of serenity from the inside out, which enhances concentration and the ability to focus your mind.

Beginner's breathing techniques

- For all breathing techniques, aim to do between five and 20 rounds (one round made up of one inhalation and one exhalation).
- Unless otherwise stated, sit in a comfortable position.
- Choose one to three techniques to include in a session.
All breathing is through the nose, unless otherwise stated.

Advanced breathing techniques

These should only be practised when you have had at least one year of experience in Yoga breathing techniques for beginners.

SUMMARY

Beginner's breathing techniques
- Sectional breathing
- Ujjayi breath
- Sithali
- Sitkari
- Brahmari
- Simhasana
- Anuloma Viloma
- Ohm

Advanced breathing techniques
- Nadhi Sodhana
- Kapalabhati
- Bandhas – Jalandhara Bandha, Moola Bandha and Uddhiyana Bandha

Do not practise any breath retention if:
- you are pregnant
- you suffer from any of the abovementioned conditions
- you are a beginner at Yoga.

General cautions
- Any breathing technique should first be learned under the guidance of an experienced teacher.

- If you feel any kind of discomfort or symptom arising as you do the practices, such as dizziness or nausea, lie down and relax in Savasana or the Child's pose for a few recovery breaths.
- Pranayama is advised after the lungs and body have been warmed and strengthened by Yoga practice. Breathing practices are best applied in the middle of a session or at the end, just before relaxation practice and meditation.

BEGINNER'S BREATHING TECHNIQUES
Sectional breathing

This technique helps to bring your attention to the three regions of breath that make up a Full Yogic Breath. It increases your lung capacity and encourages fuller breathing into the lungs. It has a deeply calming effect that replenishes the oxygen supply in the body and leads to increased energy levels and a sense of vitality. This technique is useful to include in your Yoga session to tone the respiratory muscles and help you relax in times of tension. Even taking four or five deep breaths will be effective and the Full Yogic Breath used at night (try 10 rounds) can help you to fall asleep more easily. You can also apply the Full Yogic Breath to other breathing practices, such as the Ujjayi Breath.

Start in Savasana

1. **Section 1 – Breathing into the lower region of the lung**
   Place your fingers on either side of your navel, with your elbows resting on the ground at your sides. Take three to six breaths into this area, feeling your abdomen rising and falling beneath your hands.

2. **Section 2 – Breathing into the middle region of the lung**
   Place your hands on either side of your ribcage. Take three to six breaths, feeling your ribcage expanding sideways as you inhale, moving your hands further apart. Relax on exhalation.

3. **Section 3 – Breathing into the upper region of the lung**
   Place your fingers underneath your collar bones. As you inhale, feel your upper chest rise. Try not to raise your shoulders as you inhale; keep them relaxed. As you exhale, feel the upper chest area relax.

The Full Yogic Breath

Place your arms at your sides, palms facing up. In a single inhalation, draw the air into the abdomen, then into the ribcage and into the top of the chest. On exhalation, relax the air out. Keep the in- and exhalations of equal length or lengthen the exhalation to enhance the relaxation effect.

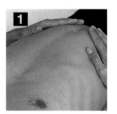 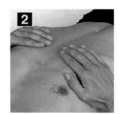 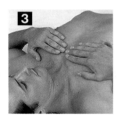

UJJAYI BREATH
The Victorious Breath

This technique helps increase lung capacity, energy levels and a state of calmness and mental clarity. The Ujjayi Breath has a soothing quality, as the sound vibration seems to massage the base of your brain.

- Sit in a comfortable position or lie down in Savasana.
- Partially close the epiglottis, which covers the windpipe at the back of the throat, so that as you inhale and exhale, the air passes through a narrower air passage, creating a soothing sound as made in deep sleep. The Ujjayi Breath creates an extended '*hhhh*' sound in the back of your throat, with your lips closed.
- To start with, keep your inhalations and exhalations even and imagine the breath following a curved or circular shape, inhaling up, then slowly allowing the breath to roll over into the exhalation. There is a natural pause at the end of each exhalation, as you let go of your breath and await the natural start of the next inhalation.
- When you find an even, natural rhythm to your breathing, begin to lengthen the exhalation, so that your exhalation aims to double the length of your inhalation. This enhances the calming effect and can help to lower blood pressure.
- If you suffer from low blood pressure, replace the lengthened exhalation with a slightly lengthened inhalation – this will raise the blood pressure.
- If this breathing does not feel comfortable, remain with even, regular breathing.

SITHALI AND SITKARI
The Cooling Breaths

The Cooling Breaths are useful in the hot months of the year. They also calm the nervous system, alleviate the symptoms of asthma and nausea and appease hunger and thirst.

Sithali

Sithali focuses on lengthening the inhalation. If this is contra-indicated for you (p150), practice with an evenly timed inhalation and exhalation or choose a technique that emphasizes the exhalation.

1. Curl your tongue, so that the sides fold up, forming a tube. Allow your tongue to protrude from your lips. Raise your chin as you inhale through your tongue (like a straw), feeling the cool air as it passes over your tongue.
2. Slightly lower your chin as you exhale through your nose, folding the tip of your tongue behind your front teeth, placing it against the palate. Repeat.
   If you are unable to curl your tongue, use Sitkari instead.

Sitkari

3. Part your jaw slightly with your tongue resting at the base of your mouth and the corners of your mouth opened out as if in a smile. Inhale and exhale through your teeth, making a hissing sound as the air passes through your teeth and over your tongue. As with Sithali, this air feels cool over the surface of your tongue.

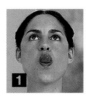 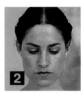

BRAHMARI
The Bee Breath

The Bee Breath lengthens the exhalation and should be practised with care (or avoided) if this is contra-indicated for you. Brahmari is said to generate joyous feelings throughout the body. It helps to clear and strengthen the respiratory system and improve vocal resonance. It has a calming and soothing effect on the body, clears and invigorates the mind and uplifts the spirit.

- With your lips closed, inhale.
- Hum as you exhale, keeping your lips closed and trying to extend the exhalation as long as possible. Use your abdominal muscles to help your breath control on exhalation. Repeat.

- If you wish to stimulate your lung cells and invigorate mind and body, tap your chest with your fists or fingers on exhalation.

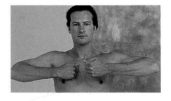

SIMHASANA
The Lion

This breath offers effective relief for a sore throat and is helpful in relieving many respiratory ailments.

- Sit on your haunches, with your hands on your thighs and your back upright.
- Inhale deeply, then exhale, opening your mouth wide, stretching your tongue out of your mouth.
  Squint to look at the point between your brow, while stretching your arms and spreading your fingers over your knees.

- Inhale and exhale two to five times, feeling your breath in the back of your throat. Exhale and return to starting position.

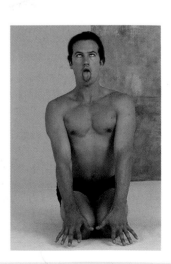

ANULOMA VILOMA
Alternate Nostril Breathing

This breathing technique helps to balance and harmonize the functioning of the right and left hemispheres of the brain. Anuloma Viloma soothes the nervous system and calms the mind. This technique is a preparation for the more advanced practise of Nadhi Sodhana.

1. Raise your right hand, curling your forefinger and middle finger into your palm, leaving your thumb, fourth finger and little finger extended.
2. Place your thumb on the right side of your nose and apply a gentle pressure at a level just under the bone, where the fleshy part of the nose begins. Inhale through the left nostril. Release and exhale through both nostrils.
3. Using your fourth finger this time, apply a gentle pressure to the left nostril, at the same level as used by the thumb on the right nostril. Inhale through your right nostril. Release and exhale through both nostrils. Repeat.

Practise with an equal length inhalation and exhalation, aiming to extend the exhalation for an enhanced purification effect (unless increasing the exhalation is contra-indicated for you).

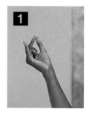 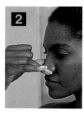 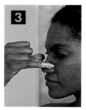

THE OHM SOUND

The Ohm sound is said to be 'the sound from which all sound originates'. Even at the quietest times of day there is never absolute silence. There is always an undercurrent of sound that resembles that of a soft breeze or the ocean in the distance. This undercurrent has been called the Ohm sound, which helps us to feel our connectedness to our environment and all that exists in the world. Repeating the Ohm sound brings peace and serenity to the mind, and by helping us tune in to the ever-present vibration, it cultivates a feeling of oneness and peace with our surroundings and the world.

The Ohm sound focuses on lengthening the exhalation when used vocally or silently with the breath.

When silently repeated in the mind, as can be helpful for meditation, the Ohm sound can be repeated on an evenly timed inhalation and exhalation.

Sit in a comfortable position. Inhale through your nose. Exhale as you vocalize the Ohm sound once, slowly. Toward the end of the exhalation, engage your abdominal muscles to assist in lengthening the exhalation. Repeat.

ADVANCED BREATHING TECHNIQUES

These practices have a powerful detoxification effect on the organs such as the liver. Discontinue your practice if any discomfort arises, and resume practice only under supervision.

NADHI SODHANA

This should only be practiced when you have enough practice in Anuloma Viloma. The hand position is as for the latter.
- Inhale through the left nostril, then exhale through the right.
- Without changing the position of the fingers, inhale through the right nostril and then change to the thumb to exhale through the left nostril. You have now completed one round.

- Continue for five to 20 rounds. If your hand gets tired during the practice, change hands.
- If you are an advanced practitioner, practise breath retention after the inhalation, using an inhalation : retention : exhalation ratio of 2 : 2 : 4 or up to 2 : 8 : 4, depending on your lung capacity and without straining.

KAPALABHATI

'Kapala' means 'skull' and 'bhati' means 'light'. This breathing practice brings light to the head area and clears the mind. Kapalabhati is a cleansing breath, involving a forced exhalation in which the abdominal muscles are quickly contracted, causing the diaphragm to push upward into the lungs. This helps the lungs to expel more stale air and carbon dioxide. Kapalabhati prepares the abdominal muscles for the Uddhiyana Bandha.

1. Kapalabhati involves a deeper inhalation because the abdomen is relaxed.
2. This is followed by a quick, active exhalation in which the abdominal muscles are contracted in toward the spine. Let go of the abdominal muscles immediately after the exhalation, so that there is a natural recoiling action of the abdominal muscles – this causes the inhalation to follow naturally. This pumping action strengthens and tones these particular muscles.

Maintain the length of your spine on the exhalation and don't involve the shoulders. After completing a round of about 20 breaths, hold the breath for a comfortable period.

- Begin with two or three relaxed deep breaths all the way down into the abdomen.
- Move on to Kapalabhati, working toward 20 rounds (a round consists of one inhalation and one exhalation).
- Once you have completed the rounds, inhale and exhale deeply, then inhale deeply once again and contract the abdomen as for Kapalabhati, holding the breath for as long as you can, without straining.
- Exhale fully and take a few relaxed breaths.
- Repeat this cycle two or three times and with practise you will find that you are able to increase the number of breaths in a cycle, to 40 or even 60 breaths.

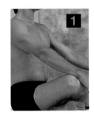 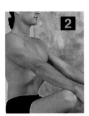

THE THREE MAIN BANDHAS
Energy seals or directors

After you have gained at least six months of experience in breathing techniques such as Ujjayi, Kapalabhati and Nadhi Sodhana, with the practise of breath retention and experience in the Yoga postures, begin to work with the bandhas. The bandhas seal in the Prana or subtle energy in the body that has been accumulated during the practise of postures and breathing. They redirect this energy to be used in nourishing the tissues and vital organs of your body; the effects may be noticed in increased energy levels and a general sense of vitality. The regular practise of bandhas rejuvenates the body and mind and helps preserve youthfulness.

The bandhas are applied while retaining the breath. Generally, Jalandhara and Moola Bandha are applied on a held inhalation and Uddhiyana Bandha is applied on a held exhalation. Only retain your breath for as long as you feel comfortable without straining. In time you will improve and be able to retain your breath for a longer period of time.

Repeat the bandhas six to 10 times, retaining your breath each time for as long as is comfortable. Then take a few deep and even recovery breaths.

It is important to learn these techniques under the supervision of an experienced teacher.

Jalandhara Bandha
A. At the start of a retained inhalation, press your chin into your chest.

Moola (or Mula) Bandha
At the start of a retained inhalation, contract your perineum (the pelvic floor muscles).

Uddhiyana Bandha
B. At the start of a retained exhalation, contract your abdominals, pulling them back and under your ribcage.

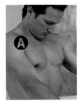

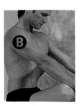

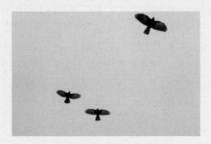

The Yoga journey

Yoga is a system of personal growth and development

– it is a lifelong journey, not a destination.

So don't expect to achieve mastery of all the Yoga postures (or even any

of them). The idea is to work toward mastery of those postures you can

comfortably achieve, without straining. Regard the photographs of the

final postures as inspiration, not intimidation.

Trust in the intelligence of your body to guide your practice, so that you can

enjoy it and reap the rewards. Maximum benefits are gained by staying true to

the level you are at and by keeping up a regular practice. Be patient with

yourself in relation to your sense of balance, your flexibility and your strength –

these will improve in time.

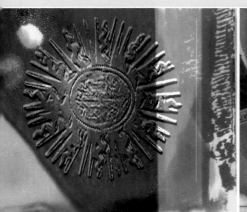
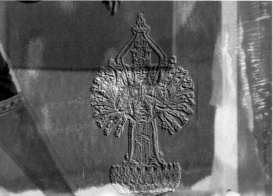
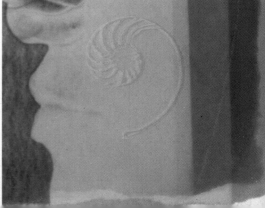

INDEX

Note: page numbers in italics refer to illustrated material.

Publishers' acknowledgements

The Publishers thank Yoga practitioners Jennifer Stephens and Henry Crafford, as well as author Noa Belling for serving as models; Yoga teacher David Jacobs for his guidance and help; hair stylist and make-up artist Dulcie Beebe for her patience, and Sumetee Pahwa for providing the Sanskrit translations and calligraphy.

Photographic credit

Yael van der Heyden, p157